THE THIRD EYE

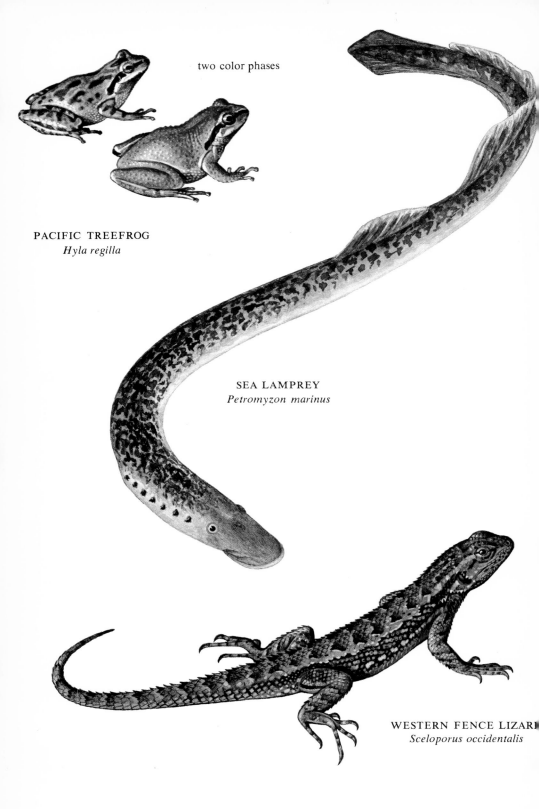

two color phases

PACIFIC TREEFROG
Hyla regilla

SEA LAMPREY
Petromyzon marinus

WESTERN FENCE LIZARD
Sceloporus occidentalis

The Third Eye, *1973.*

Richard M. Eakin

University of California Press
Berkeley · Los Angeles · London

University of California Press
Berkeley and Los Angeles, California
University of California Press, Ltd.
London, England

Copyright © 1973, by
The Regents of the University of California
ISBN: 0–520–02413–3
Library of Congress Catalog Card Number: 72–97740
Printed in the United States of America
Designed by Jean Peters

To the state and federal taxpayer who supported my scientific studies through the University of California and the United States Public Health Service.

Contents

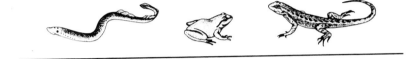

Preface

Third eyes have long excited the imaginations of storytellers and the curiosity of biologists. The reader will recall the giant cyclops Polyphemus in Homer's *Odyssey* and the three sisters (One-Eye, Two-Eyes, and Three-Eyes) in Grimms' *Fairy Tales*. In the instance of Polyphemus and Sister One-Eye, the single median eye was probably a developmental anomaly resulting from the fusion of the primordia of the lateral eyes in an early embryonic stage. Neither Homer nor Brothers Grimm appear to have known this biological explanation. Sister Three-Eyes, however, had in addition to her lateral eyes a third one in the center of the forehead. The third eye was not, I am very sure, an embryonic mistake, a cyclopian eye, but a pineal eye, the kind I shall discuss in this book. It must have been a remarkable (also Grimm) throwback to the third eye of our reptilian ancestors.

Scientific interest in third eyes began just one hundred years ago, with the discovery of the pineal or parietal eye in a lizard by Franz Leydig (1872). The present work is therefore a centennial commemorative. Its genesis was an article in the *American Scientist* (Eakin, 1970) entitled "A Third Eye." I received positive feedback from readers on the light style used in that paper, which might have been titled "*Sceloporus* and I" (*Sceloporus* is the scientific [generic] name of the fence lizard whose third eye I have studied). I was further stimulated to be informal upon receiving the following limerick from a dear aunt, Annie Simminger, of Manteca, California.

In Berkeley there once lived a wizard
Who studied the eyes of a lizard.
When he found there were three
He danced and cried, "Whee-e-e-e!
I'll now take a look at his gizzard!"

I have endeavored to use nontechnical language as much as possible either by omitting professional terminology or by placing it in parentheses, in the hope that my story will be read by those with limited educations in biology. Although scientific terms are intended to give precision, often they dull the general reader's interest and fetter his understanding. I beg the patience of the sophisticated professional who samples these pages. Last, to the many investigators in pineal photobiology whose works have not been cited I offer my apologies. I have drawn heavily upon the Californian studies in the interest of giving a personal account. Much research has been undertaken this year to verify earlier conclusions, to obtain missing information on the anatomy and development of third eyes, and to procure better or fresh illustrations.

Many friends have contributed to the creation of this work. I am especially grateful to the following: Jean Leutwiler Brandenburger, talented and gracious research associate for many years, who participated in most aspects of the project; Millie Miller Ferlatte, devoted research assistant, and her successor, Carol Mortensen, for preparation of the figures for publication (additionally, Mrs. Ferlatte assisted in the new studies on third eyes mentioned above); Emily E. Reid, departmental artist, for transforming my sketches into finished drawings and for the painting of the lamprey in the frontispiece; Victor C. Duran and Alfred A. Blaker, University Scientific Photographers, who made the light micrographs and the photographs of the characters in the story; Merianne O'Grady and Teriann Asami for producing the ribbon copy of the manuscript and making the index; Judith Quinn for editing the manuscript; Jean Peters for designing the book; Drs. Jean-Pierre Collin, Eberhard Dodt, Duco I. Hamasaki, David S. McDevitt, William H. Miller, Myron L. Wolbarsht, Fred D. Warner, and Richard W. Young for certain figures identified in the accompanying legends; and the following biologists, who advised me variously—Drs. Collin, Dodt, Hamasaki, Gerald P. Cooper, William I. Follett, Douglas E. Kelly, Wilbur B. Quay, and especially Robert C. Stebbins, to whom I am additionally indebted for my interest in pineal eyes and for the use in the frontispiece of three of his beautiful paintings.* Finally, I value the assistance of certain critics, unknown to me, who read an unpolished draft of this essay and advised the University of California Press of its merits and weaknesses.

I acknowledge the bibliographic help of the Brain Information Service of the University of California, Los Angeles, the courtesy of several publishers for permission to reproduce copyrighted illustrations, and the excellent craftsmanship of the University of California Press. And I am profoundly grateful to the United States Public Health Service for a grant-in-aid (GM 10292) for the past ten years and for financial assistance in the publication of this book and to my alma mater, the University of California, which has nurtured me and then sustained me throughout my professional career, and which generously provided a sabbatical leave to produce this work.

R. M. E.

* From Reptiles and Amphibians of the San Francisco Bay Region by Robert C. Stebbins, University of California Press, 1959.

1
Dramatis Personae

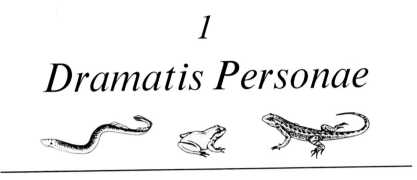

The Western Fence Lizard (Sceloporus occidentalis)

This animal, known to youthful collectors as a blue-belly, was selected to be the leading character of my story because it has one of
the best third eyes known. When I studied freshman zoology, however, I was introduced to the third eye as the unique possession of a
celebrated New Zealand reptile, *Sphenodon* (from two Greek words:
spheno, meaning 'wedge,' and *dont*, 'tooth'). The textbook stated that
this feature, among others, entitled *Sphenodon* to be called a living
fossil. The animal is also known by its Maori name, Tuatara (from
the native word *tua*, meaning 'back side,' and *tara*, 'spine'). When,
many years later, my colleague Robert C. Stebbins persuaded me to
take an active interest in the reptilian third eye, I learned to my surprise that our local fence lizard had an even better third eye than that
of *Sphenodon*. Therewith vanished a good excuse for a trip to that
zoological wonderland, the home of not only the tuatara, but of peri-
patus, the kiwi, and the glowworm. Now, after fifteen years of off-
and-on study of *Sceloporus occidentalis*, I am considerably enlight-
ened about its median eye and also its behavior. My knowledge of the
latter was acquired not through planned research but from many
hours of patiently stalking blue-bellies in the field with a fishing pole
to whose tip was tied a noose of copper wire (Eakin, 1957). I have
come to regard the Western Fence Lizard as a special friend. The
affection, however, is unidirectional; occasionally I am bitten, as
I should be if the lizards knew my intentions and their fate. But their

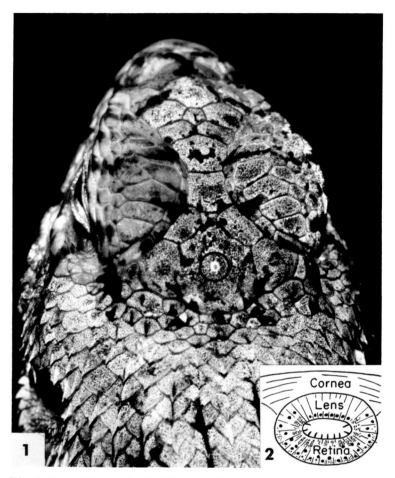

Fig. 1. Top of head of adult Western Fence Lizard (*Sceloporus occidentalis*). Third eye is white spot (encircled) beneath center of large (interparietal) scale. × 7. Heretofore unpublished, Eakin and Blaker.

Fig. 2. Sketch of cross section through third eye of *S. occidentalis*.

teeth, although sharp, are small, and they have yet to draw blood.

The third eye of *S. occidentalis* is barely visible to the unaided human eye as a yellowish spot beneath a large scale (interparietal) on the top of the head behind the level of the large lateral eyes (see Fig. 1). Because of its position in an opening (foramen) between the two parietal bones of the skull, the organ is technically termed the parietal eye. It has a diameter of only a few tenths of a millimeter. A section through it (Fig. 2) reveals the following: cornea, the overlying transparent skin; lens, a palisade of clear cells, which constitutes the roof of the eye; fluid-filled cavity; and retina, a thick layer forming the floor and sides of the eye.

The Pacific Treefrog (Hyla regilla)

The amphibian character in my cast is a small, colorful frog, widely distributed west of the Rockies and best known for its nightly choruses which lull the camper to sleep. Contrary to its name, over most of its range it is seldom found in trees! I have spent many delightful hours in search of its eggs and embryos in ponds and streams in the Berkeley hills. The specimen shown in Figure 3 does not truly belong in this story, but I had a fondness for him. I surgically removed the primordium of his pituitary gland when he was an early embryo before the onset of movement. Lacking the intermediate lobe of his master gland (and hence its melanophore-stimulating hormone, essential for normal pigmentation), he became a silvery tadpole that under loving care transformed into this beautiful creature, the likes of which one does not find naturally.

Now, the adult Pacific Treefrog is unusual, as most frogs go, in that it lacks a third eye, but it possesses a good one as a tadpole, upon which all of my study of the amphibian eye has been conducted. In the larva of this form and in the adults of other species the organ is situated on top of the head, far forward in the midline at the level of the front (anterior) margins of the lateral eyes. Its position is marked by a circle on the photograph of my albino frog (Fig. 3). When the eye is present, the overlying skin is transparent, owing to the absence of pigment cells. The clearing is called the brow spot. The eye is more properly termed the frontal organ because of its position between the frontal bones of the skull and because it does not appear eyelike. The first describer, the German anatomist Alfred Stieda, called it a *Stirndrüse* ('forehead gland') or *Stirnorgan* ('forehead organ') because he thought that it must be some kind of glandular structure.

The frontal organ is a small body (Fig. 4) about one- or two-tenths of a millimeter in its greatest dimension. Its shape is variable:

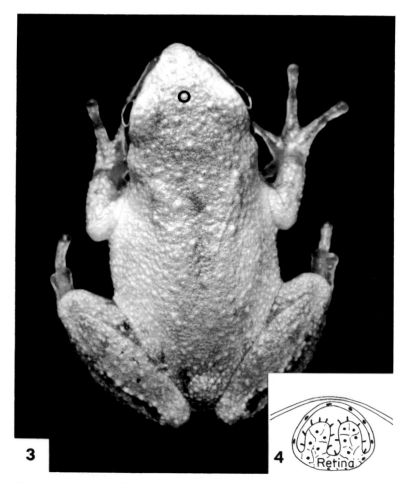

Fig. 3. Subadult Pacific Treefrog (*Hyla regilla*). Circle on top of head indicates position of third eye (frontal organ) in larval stage of this frog and in adults of certain other frogs. × 9. From Eakin and Bush (1957).

Fig. 4. Sketch of cross section of frontal organ in tadpole of *H. regilla*.

spherical, oval, pearlike. Unlike the third eye of a lizard, the amphibian frontal organ has no lens, its upper wall being a thin layer of cells. The cavity of the organ is irregular and inconstant. There is usually a principal chamber and one or more extensions of it into the floor of the retina, which is simply a mound of cells. Not much of an eye, one might say—certainly inferior to the parietal eye of *Sceloporus* in general form and structure. But, as I shall discuss later, it transforms the light energy which it receives through the brow spot into nervous messages.

The Pacific Lamprey (Entosphenus tridentatus)*

The third member of my cast was chosen for two reasons. It represents the lowest forms of living vertebrates, the cyclostomes, which are jawless, limbless creatures of great evolutionary significance. Second, it has not one but two third eyes. They, like the amphibian frontal organ, are situated forward on the midline of the head (Fig. 5) beneath a transparent area of skin. My study of the lamprey's third eyes has been limited to the larval form, called the ammocoetes (from two Greek words: *ammo*, meaning 'sand,' and *koite*, 'bed'). Ammocoetes live in the sandy banks of streams. The adults come from the sea annually, like salmon, to spawn in the gravel beds of our coastal rivers and then die. Upon hatching, the young ammocoetes burrow in the sand. They feed on debris and microscopic organisms, which they filter from the water as it passes through the mouth and out the gill slits. After several years of this mode of existence the ammocoetes, now six inches or more in length, transform (metamorphose) into adult lampreys which migrate to the sea, where they live as parasites on fishes. Because of the marked differences in structure and behavior between larval and adult stages, the ammocoetes was once thought to be a separate species of animal and was so classified by zoologists.

The two third eyes are sacs, or vesicles, not unlike the amphibian frontal organ, one on top of the other (Fig. 6). The upper (dorsal) one is called a pineal eye because it is an extension of the pineal body (epiphysis) that is situated farther back (posterior) on the surface of the brain. The lower one is a parietal organ because it is developmentally similar (homologous) to the parietal eye of lizards, as we

---

* The Sea Lamprey (*Petromyzon marinus*) was used in some of my studies, and it was chosen instead of *Entosphenus tridentatus* for the frontispiece because it is more colorful than its west coast relative.

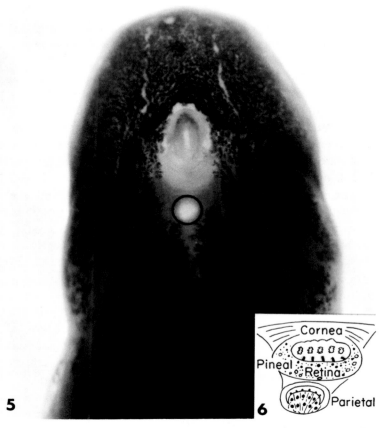

5

6

Fig. 5. Top of head of young ammocoetes of Pacific Lamprey (*Entosphenus tridentatus*). Pineal and parietal eyes (encircled) lie beneath clear area of skin. Median nasal opening situated anterior to third eyes. × 12. Heretofore unpublished, Eakin and Blaker.

Fig. 6. Sketch of cross section through pineal eye (above) and parietal eye (below) of *E. tridentatus.*

shall discuss later. There is a little asymmetry in the position of the two vesicles: the pineal one is slightly to the right, the parietal one to the left—a point of evolutionary importance. The organs are alike in having relatively thin roofs and thick retinal floors; the cavity of the pineal eye is spacious, but that of the parietal vesicle is narrow and arched.

The Universal Cilium (Cilium ubiquitum)

I fancy the reader exclaiming: "Wait a minute. How silly can you be? You mean that a cilium is a character in this book? That little vibrating hair, legions of which line our windpipes and cover the bodies of many microscopic organisms?" "Of course," I reply, "Why not? True, it is not an animal,—only a minute part of one—but it plays an indispensable role in the function not only of third eyes but of lateral eyes, also. In fact, for many animals vision without cilia would be impossible, and, I might add, hearing and smelling and certain other senses. But these cilia differ from those of the windpipe in being nonmotile and in being specialized for reception of light energy (photons)."

A motile cilium (kinocilium) is a long, cylindrical shaft (Fig. 7) within which lies a remarkable locomotor apparatus (axoneme) composed of fine tubes, called microtubules, observable only with an electron microscope. The microtubules are arranged in a bundle extending the length of the cilium in a specific pattern, best shown by a cross section (Fig. 8). A ring of nine pairs of microtubules (doublets) lies beneath the ciliary membrane and encloses two central microtubules (singlets). This pattern is called $9 \times 2 + 2$. One of the tubules in each doublet possesses a pair of arms composed of a protein (named dynein by Professor Ian Gibbons of the University of Hawaii, see Gibbons, 1965) which is an enzyme (ATPase) that probably implements the movement of the cilium. A current theory of ciliary action advanced by my colleague Peter Satir (1967) holds that a sliding of the microtubular doublets upon one another produces a bending of the cilium that sweeps the length of its shaft. A discussion of this theory has been published recently by Charles J. Brokaw (1972). Waves of many cilia, beating in concert, serve organisms in various ways—to move them through a liquid or to circulate fluids within their bodies or to transport particles and cells. Familiar examples are the swimming of microscopic organisms in the sea or fresh-water lakes and streams; the move-

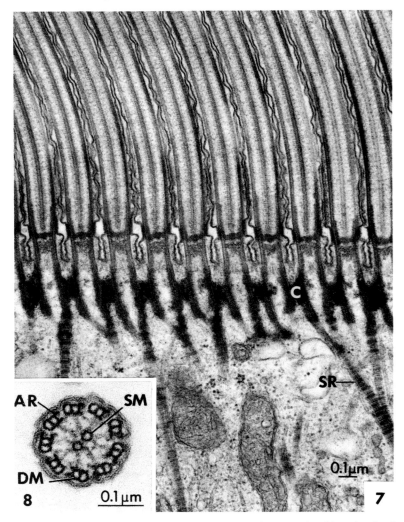

Fig. 7. Electron micrograph (hereafter abbreviated EM) of longitudinal section through several motile cilia from gill of a clam (*Elliptio complanatus*). C, centriole (kinetosome or basal body); SR, striated rootlet. × 50,000.

Fig. 8. EM of cross section of a cilium from gill of *E. complanatus*. AR, arm on one microtubule of a doublet; DM, doublet of microtubules; SM, single microtubule. Arms on microtubules intensified by retouching. × 120,000. Figs. 7 and 8 courtesy of Dr. Fred D. Warner.

ment of flatworms over rocks and plants; the transport of eggs and sperm along ciliated reproductive ducts, aided in the instance of the sperm by their own cilia (flagella); and removal of foreign particles from respiratory passages or the wafting of food particles into a mouth.

Sensory cilia, by contrast to motile ones, are modified in at least two respects: they lack the central singlets of microtubules (hence, $9 \times 2 + 0$) and also the arms on each doublet. Their nonmotility is probably a consequence of the absence of these structures, especially the enzyme-containing arms. Additionally, light-sensitive cilia have evolved some kind of membranous apparatus for capturing radiant energy. In the instance of photoreceptors of vertebrates (that is, the light-absorbing cilia in median and lateral eyes) the ciliary membrane is evaginated serially to give an amazing stack of disks which require an electron microscope to be seen. The disks in a third-eye receptor are shown in the electron micrograph (a photograph made with an electron microscope) reproduced as Figure 9. It is hard to believe that this orderly array of units was produced by a smooth membrane on the surface of a cylindrical cilium. The reader will observe that the disks (D) are attached to the shaft (SH) of the cilium (to the left) and that in this shaft there are microtubules (MT_1), one of which may be seen connected basally to a dark cylinder called a centriole (C_1). If one took a cross section of a sensory cilium above its centriole, one would behold the full constellation of microtubules in their beautiful $9 \times 2 + 0$ pattern (Fig. 10). The centriole is likewise composed of a ring of nine units of microtubules. The units are not doublets, however, but triplets (Fig. 11). One more detail at this time—adjacent to the centriole on the reader's right is a circular structure. This is another centriole (C_2), an accessory one, which is cut transversely owing to its usual position at right angles to the primary centriole. The accessory centriole is also a short cylinder composed of nine triplets of microtubules (not observable in Fig. 9).

In the first lecture each year in my course in general zoology I endeavor to pique the students' interest in a formal study of animals, including man, by describing some features of the living world which have been exciting to me. This I do, not because I have anything profound to give, but because personal experience appears to

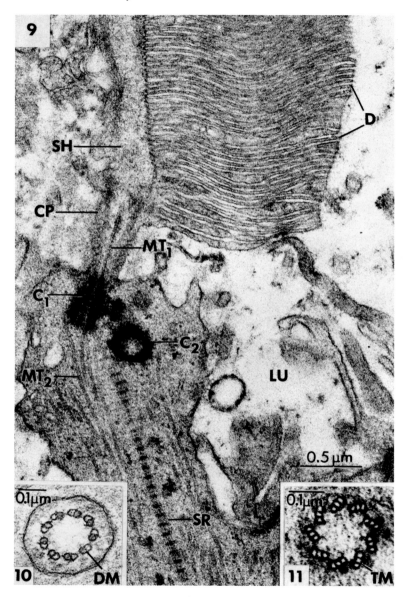

have more impact than quotations from great biologists, unless, of course, one impersonates them with costumes and makeup. Two of my points are the continuity and diversity in nature. I use cilia to illustrate both. Cilia may be found in all major groups of animals (phyla) and in most of those in the plant kingdom. Moreover, from organisms which are neither plant nor animal (protists) up to the ginkgo tree and man, cilia are remarkably alike. The $9 \times 2 + 2$ pattern of microtubules is omnipresent. There must be something unique, and indispensable about this architecture which explains its persistence. Cilia illustrate the profound continuity in organisms, as do mitochondria, the structures which transfer energy within cells, and as do the four molecules composing the genetic code. At the same time nature has modified the cilium in remarkable ways to serve functions other than locomotion. One variation, the sensory cilium in a third eye, has just been introduced. In Chapter 2 I shall describe other kinds of photoreceptoral cilia, and there are still other examples of diversification of cilia which lie beyond the bounds of this book. And so the cilium has through eons retained certain basic features, but at the same time it has exhibited great plasticity, especially in its membrane and in the evolution of disks, villi, lamellae, and tubules for sensory perception. It illustrates the Darwinian principle of descent with modification.

Then I endeavor to apply that principle to the alleged paragon of evolution, man, and to his future and that of the world he dominates. When I return to teaching after writing this book, my comments will reflect the impact of a recent reading of some essays in honor of Erich Fromm, particularly those of George Wald, Loren Eiseley, and Theodosius Dobzhansky (see Landis and Tauber, 1971).

Fig. 9. EM of longitudinal section of photoreceptoral cilium from parietal eye of *S. occidentalis*. c_1, distal centriole (kinetosome); c_2, accessory or proximal centriole; CP, connecting piece; D, disks in outer segment of receptoral process; LU, lumen of eye; MT_1, microtubule of cilium; MT_2, microtubule in inner segment of receptoral process; SH, shaft of cilium; SR, striated rootlet. $\times$ 33,000. Heretofore unpublished, Eakin and Brandenburger.

Figs. 10 and 11. EM of cross sections of, respectively, connecting piece and distal centriole of photoreceptor in parietal eye of *S. occidentalis*. DM, doublet of microtubules; TM, triplet of microtubules. $\times$ 74,000 (Fig. 10); $\times$ 89,000 (Fig. 11). Fig. 10 from Eakin (1968); Fig. 11, heretofore unpublished, Eakin and Brandenburger.

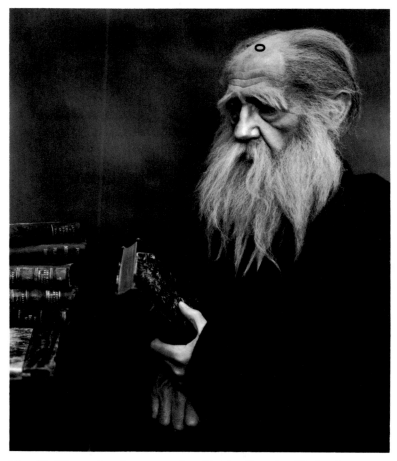

Fig. 12. The author impersonating Charles Darwin. Circle above fore-head indicates presumed position of third eye if *Homo sapiens* had one. Alfred A. Blaker, photographer.

The Author (Homo sapiens)

The first person singular is used so frequently in this book that I am immodestly entering my name on the list of characters even though I do not have a third eye (Fig. 12). I wish, however, that third eyes had not been lost in the evolution of mammals from their reptilian ancestors. How useful they might be to monitor the sky for falling objects or to observe passersby while pretending to doze in a city park!

2
Evolution

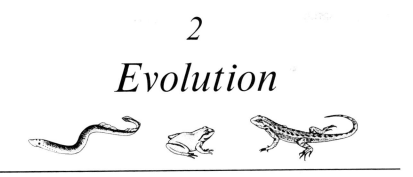

When did nature invent the third eye? Were there prevertebrate antecedents? How large was the eye in ancient amphibians and reptiles? Was it ever paired? And why was it lost in the evolution of birds and mammals? These are examples of questions to lay before a pineal historian, one of the best of whom was the late Tilly Edinger at the Museum of Comparative Zoology, Harvard University.

History of a Foramen

Third eyes have not been preserved in any known fossil vertebrate, but their presence in the past is indicated by a hole, the parietal or pineal foramen, on the top of the skull of extinct fishes, amphibians, and reptiles. Figure 13 illustrates the parietal foramen in the leading character of our story, *Sceloporus occidentalis*. The specimen was a young adult male collected by Dr. Stebbins on a field trip which we made to Forty-nine Palms in southern California many years ago. The foramen measures 1.1 mm in diameter. One of the largest parietal openings (2×3 mm) in a contemporary lizard is that of the giant monitor, the Komodo lizard (*Varanus komodoensis*) of Ceylon. The parietal foramen was much larger, however, in many fossil reptiles. In one form (a Permian cotylosaur) it was 15 by 28 mm (see Edinger, 1955). But can one assume that the foramen in the skull of an ancient reptile once contained an eye? And if so, can one assume that there is a correlation between the size of the foramen and the size of the third eye?

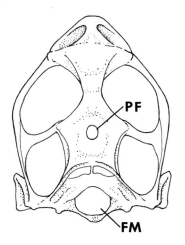

Fig. 13. Sketch of top of skull of *S. oc-cidentalis.* FM, foramen magnum; PF, parietal or pineal foramen. × 4. Heretofore unpublished. Emily E. Reid, delineator.

The major argument against the presumption that a median aperture on the top of a fossil skull accommodated an eye is that the foramen was inconstant in position, being situated forward near the nasal openings in some forms and near the hind end of the cranium in others. This means, of course, that the bones surrounding the foramen were not the same in all fossils. In the language of the embryologist and anatomist, the foramina are nonhomologous. As I read the paleontologists, however, there seems to be a consensus that the foramina did indeed contain pineal sense organs. Dr. Edinger stated: "If one doubts an association of a parietal foramen with a parietal eye one may as well doubt that the orbits of fossil skulls contained lateral eyes" (Edinger, 1955). Jarvik (1967) advanced the idea that when the foramen was far forward (for example, at the anterior border of the frontal bones), it accommodated a pineal eye, and when situated in the rear (for example, in the suture between frontals and parietals or between the parietals), it held a parietal eye. A more fundamental distinction between pineal and parietal will be given later.

Dr. Edinger made a strong case for the validity of the assumption that a large parietal foramen held a large third eye. She analyzed the literature and found a good correspondence in modern lizards between the size of the parietal foramen and that of the third eye. Specimens in which there was a significant discrepancy were thought to be juveniles. This explanation is supported by my experience in removing parietal eyes from *Sceloporus*: the foramen in young blue-bellies is large, whereas that of old adults is small—a little larger than the eye and its capsule. Dr. Edinger (1955) concluded, "In my opinion the size relations between foramen and eye in extant lizards entitle the paleontologist to conclude that the larger the parietal foramen in a fossil skull, the larger was the organ it served."

But the reader may point out that ancient reptiles were usually giants in comparison with lizards living today, and one would expect large parietal foramina in them. We should not compare absolute dimensions of the foramina, however, but the relationship between the size of the parietal foramen and that of some other feature of the skull. Dr. Edinger did just that. She compared the parietal foramen of each specimen with its foramen magnum, the hole at the posterior end of the cranium through which the spinal cord passes. In most contemporary lizards the former is about a fifth to a third the size of the latter. In most fossil reptiles, on the other hand, the two apertures were about the same size; in some, probably specialized species, the parietal foramen was even larger than the foramen magnum. In the oldest reptile known, *Seymouria*, the parietal foramen was only one-third to a half the size of the foramen magnum, but the pineal opening was cone-shaped, its internal diameter being half again as large as its outer diameter. This stout, short-tailed creature, about twenty inches in length, lived around 280 million years ago (lower Permian period) and was so similar to an amphibian that its assignment to the class Reptilia or to the class Amphibia is a matter of opinion. According to Professor A. S. Romer, one of our best authorities on vertebrate evolution: "*Seymouria* seems to stand almost exactly on the dividing line between amphibians and reptiles. . . . The distinction between them is fundamentally one of modes of development. Did *Seymouria* lay its eggs? Probably this question will never be answered" (1945).

From *Seymouria* it is an easy step back in time to the ancient amphibians which also had pineal foramina on the tops of their heads. But they were not so large as that of *Seymouria* and were small in comparison with that of later reptiles. Why? A mystery writer does not usually reveal his secret in the second chapter, but perhaps it would be useful at this point to give a hint of the ultimate objective of this essay, to develop the theory of function of the third eye suggested by Dr. Stebbins and me in our first paper (Stebbins and Eakin, 1958). We proposed that the organ serves an animal, such as *Sceloporus,* as a dosimeter of solar radiation. The information gained thereby is used, along with input from other light-sensitive structures (photoreceptors) in regulating the daily cycle of activities (circadian rhythm) of the lizard. I shall expand on this concept in Chapter 5. In line with this theory, a well-developed third eye fully exposed by a large foramen in the cranial roof seems more useful to a terrestrial animal (reptile) than to a semi-aquatic one (amphibian). I am not surprised, therefore, to learn from the paleontologist that the ancient amphibians had relatively small parietal foramina.

The foramen was present, almost without exception, in even the stem amphibians (labyrinthodonts). One of these primitive amphibians was *Eogyrinus attheyi*, a giant fish-like creature about fifteen feet long. It lived around 350 million years ago (Carboniferous period) in the lakes of the great coal forests. It used its powerful, laterally compressed tail for locomotion and for defense against large predators—sharks and lungfishes—which inhabited the same waters. When the lakes began to dry up, *Eogyrinus* probably moved on land with its short and feeble limbs in search of other pools with more water. Its pineal foramen was only 2 mm in diameter, but a third eye was surely there ready to play its role, along with limbs, lungs, and nasal passages, in the new, terrestrial way of life. The evolutionist calls this state of readiness for an evolutionary advance preadaptation. Whether the third eye of the preterrestrial vertebrate served a function is a point of speculation.

And what about ancient fishes? Yes, many of them also had parietal foramina, and, more important, in some they were paired. Tilly Edinger (1956) made a special report on paired or partly subdivided pineal apertures in fishes that swam the seas and streams between 350 and 400 million years ago (Devonian period). Some

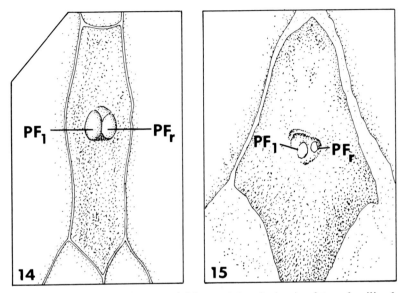

Figs. 14 and 15. Median cranial bone (pineal plate) of two fossilized ancient fishes (arthrodires)—respectively, *Pholidosteus friedeli* and *Rinosteus tuberculatus*—bearing two pineal foramina or thinnings in the bone, left and right (PF_l and PF_r). From Stensiö (1963); Emily E. Reid, delineator.

of them were jointed-necked fishes (arthrodires), some were armored sharks (stegoselachians), and still others were very early lungfishes (dipnoans). Figures 14 and 15, taken from papers by the Danish paleontologist Professor Erik Stensiö (1963), show the parietal foramina in two of these fishes. In some instances the right foramen was the larger, in others the left one. Edinger (1956) concluded, "right and left pineal sense organs were equipotential but developed unequally, both in the embryology of those ancient fishes and during the evolution of vertebrates." As noted in introducing our third character, lampreys today retain the ancestral plan of two third eyes, and, although one is superimposed on the other in the midline, there is a slight asymmetry, and they show right (pineal) and left (parietal) connections to the brain. Later I shall discuss other evidence of an early bilaterality in vertebrate third eyes.

Prevertebrate Origin

We have traced the history of third eyes as far as we can by using the paleontological record. Is our search for evolutionary origins at an end? No, there is a median eye in an organism that lives today, whose ancestry probably antedates the first vertebrates. I refer to the sea squirt, an uninspiring animal with a dirty, slimy skin and two siphons, one for intake and one for outlet of seawater, from which the organism strains food particles and absorbs oxygen. As one separates a specimen from a piling or pier, it squirts a jet of water from its excurrent siphon, hence its name. Sea squirts are also called tunicates because of the leathery tunic which encloses the vital parts, or ascidians (from the Greek work *askidion,* meaning 'little wineskin' or 'bladder').

Now, the adult sea squirt is degenerate and offers no help in our quest for the origin of the vertebrate third eye because it has no eye. In fact, one would not recognize it as a member of the most advanced group (Phylum Chordata) of the animal kingdom, to which belong the vertebrates (cyclostomes, true fishes, amphibia, reptiles, birds, and mammals), plus a few prevertebrates in addition to the tunicates. But the larva of a sea squirt is a respectable chordate, with a brain, spinal cord, gill slits, muscle segments, fins, a skeletal rod (the notochord, from which feature the phylum takes its name), and a median eye (Fig. 16). And it swims in the manner of a fish.

The eye of an ascidian tadpole (*Ciona intestinalis*), which I have studied with the assistance of Miss Aileen Kuda, is more properly designated ocellus, meaning 'little eye' or 'eyespot.' It consists of a one-celled, pigmented cup (Fig. 17) in whose cavity rests a relatively enormous lens composed of three cells. On the outside of the pigmented cup is a layer of fifteen to twenty (estimate) sensory cells.

Fig. 16. Sketch of longitudinal section through head and part of tail of an ascidian tadpole of *Ciona intestinalis.*

Fig. 17. EM of longitudinal section through ocellus of ascidian tadpole of *C. intestinalis.* GL, masses of glycogen granules; LCN, nuclei of lens cells; LM, sensory lamellae; LU, lumen of brain (cerebral vesicle); M, mitochondria; PC, cup-shaped pigmented cell; RC, sensory cells. × 6,800. From Eakin and Kuda (1971).

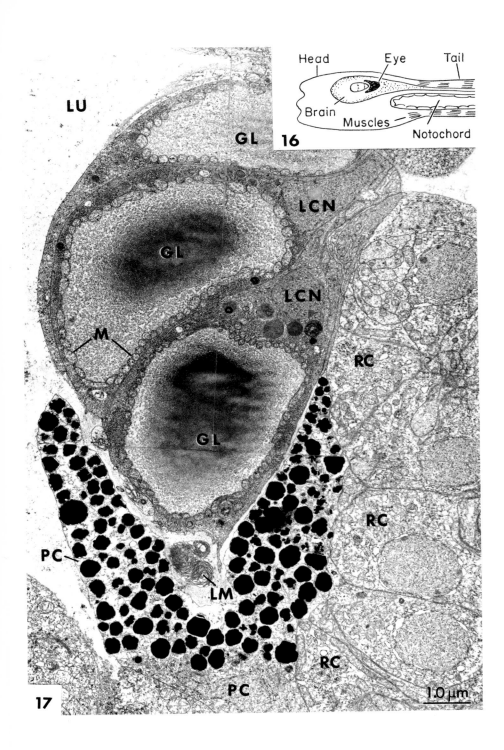

LU

GL

Head   Eye   Tail

Brain   Muscles   Notochord

16

LCN

GL

LCN

M

RC

GL

RC

PC

LM

RC

PC

17   1.0 µm

Extensions of these cells pass through folds in the pigmented cell to reach the narrow cleft between lens and eyecup, where they give rise to a stack of membranes or lamellae (LM). The British investigator Noël Dilly (1961, 1964) was the first to observe the piled membranes, for which electron microscopy is needed. He proposed that they are photoreceptoral structures and called attention to their similarity to the disks of rods and cones in the eyes of vertebrates. He even stated that they were ciliary receptors, but without having the evidence.

What is the evidence? Let our fourth character, the cilium, answer this question. Point 1: anatomists should demonstrate that the membranes are associated with a bundle of microtubules (axoneme) in a $9 \times 2 + 2$ or $9 \times 2 + 0$ pattern. Point 2: they should also find a centriole at the base of the axoneme. Miss Kuda and I obtained this evidence (Eakin and Kuda, 1971; Eakin, 1972), and we can now assert with confidence that the photoreceptors of ascidian larvae are ciliary. Our findings have been confirmed by Barnes (1971). The electron micrograph in Figure 18 shows the necks of four sensory cells (RC_1–RC_4) passing through folds in the pigmented cell (PC) and each giving rise to a stack of membranes and a bundle of microtubules (axoneme). Because the sections used in electron microscopy are so thin (from 0.06 to 0.1 of a micrometer) one cannot see all of the microtubules in one section. Two are shown in the third receptor (RC_3), and the discerning reader will note segments of four microtubules in the first cell (RC_1). In favorable cross sections (not shown) we had clear confirmation of a $9 \times 2 + 0$ pattern. At the base of each axoneme lies a centriole. The centrioles in the first three cells were cut longitudinally; that in the lowest cell (RC_4) was sectioned transversely. The magnification is too low, however, for the reader to see the nine triplets.

The light-sensitive part of each receptor is the stack of membranes (LM). They are infoldings of the ciliary membrane, giving arrays of flat plates (lamellae) parallel to the cilium (see Fig. 19). As all cilia in the ascidian ocellus lie at right angles to the long axis of the lens (Fig. 18), the lamellae are likewise perpendicular to this axis and to the direction of incoming light. The disks in third-eye receptors (see Fig. 9) and those of rods and cones of vertebrate lateral eyes, on the other hand, are at right angles to the cilium. In

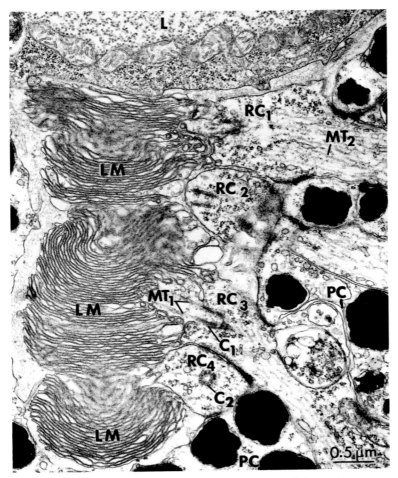

Fig. 18. EM of longitudinal section through parts of four photorecep-toral cells (RC_1–RC_4) in ocellus of tadpole of *C. intestinalis*. C_1, distal centriole (kinetosome); C_2, proximal or accessory centriole; L, lens cell (lower border of innermost lens cell); LM, lamellae of receptoral pro-cesses; MT_1, ciliary microtubules; MT_2, cytoplasmic microtubule; PC, fingers of single pigmented cell. × 19,500. From Eakin and Kuda (1971).

both ascidian and vertebrate eyes, however, the lamellae and disks are perpendicular to the direction of incoming light. The membranes of the disks and lamellae contain molecules of light-sensitive, vita-min-A–based substances called photopigments in a quasi-crystalline

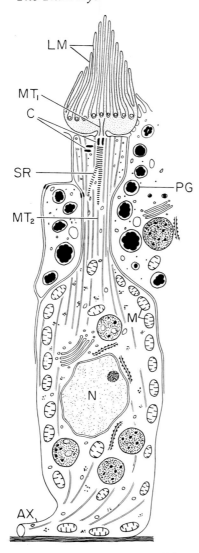

Fig. 19. Diagram of photoreceptoral cell in ocellus of *C. intestinalis*. AX, axon (nerve fiber) from sensory cell; C, centrioles (distal and proximal); LM, sensory lamellae derived from cilium; M, mitochondria; MT_1, microtubule (in axoneme of cilium); M_2, microtubule in cytoplasm; N, nucleus; PG, pigment granule; SR, striated rootlet of cilium. From Eakin and Kuda, 1971; Emily E. Reid, delineator.

pattern (Wald, Brown, and Gibbons, 1963). This orientation presumably favors the maximal absorption of radiant energy.

I admit that the suggestion of the ascidian ocellus as a forerunner of the vertebrate eye is highly speculative. The supporting arguments are: both are median; both arise from the wall of the embryonic brain (neural tube); and in both the photoreceptors are ciliary in nature, and they project from the front surface of the retina instead of from its back side, as do the rods and cones of vertebrate lateral eyes. The lenses differ, although not significantly. In the ascidian ocellus each of the three lens cells contains an enormous mass of granules (see Fig. 17), which Miss Kuda and I have shown to be composed of a complex carbohydrate, glycogen (Eakin and Kuda, 1972). The lens cells of the reptilian median eye, the only one with a lens, do not contain aggregations of glycogen. If the ascidian ocellus is the predecessor of the parietal eye, one might ask, what are the forerunners of the vertebrate lateral eyes? To this question I have no answer, as no known chordate without vertebrae possesses a pair of lateral eyes, or even eyespots.

There is one other primitive chordate, the lancelet, or amphioxus, which possesses modified cilia projecting from the roof of its brain (cerebral vesicle) into the neural cavity. These cilia have lateral, sheetlike extensions (see Eakin, 1963) similar to the lamellae of the receptors in the ascidian eye. Although this creature, which lives in the intertidal mud or sand, is exceedingly light-sensitive, there is no physiological or biochemical evidence that the cerebral cilia are indeed photoreceptoral. There are eyespots along the spinal cord of this animal which have nonciliary photoreceptors (Eakin and Westfall, 1962a) and are, therefore, clearly off the line of evolution under discussion.

History of Light-sensitive Cilia

Assuming that the ocellus of the ascidian tadpole and the membranous cilia in the dorsal wall of the brain of amphioxus foreshadowed the vertebrate third eye, what preceded them? It would be logical to look at the ancestors of the chordates. But there is no agreement among zoologists on the origin of the Phylum Chordata. We are not without theories, however. It has been suggested that our remote predecessors were segmented worms (Phylum Annelida) or creatures resembling the so-called horseshoe crabs (Phylum Arthropoda) or animals like sea stars, sea urchins, and sea cucumbers (Phylum Echinodermata) or small marine organisms with crowns of tentacles (the lophophorate phyla). Mollusks have never been seriously considered ancestral to our phylum. Although some of them have excellent eyes, such as the squid and octopus, most molluskan light receptors are fundamentally unlike the ciliary photo-receptors of chordates. The annelid and arthropod theories are, to my knowledge, without protagonists today. That leaves the echino-derms and the lophophorates. The best eye in these groups is the eyecup, or ocellus, at the tip of each arm of a sea star. It would not take much alteration to convert an echinoderm ocellus into an ascidian eye—just add a simple lens, mutate the red pigment in the eye-cup to a black one, and change the style of the cilium by transforming the villi which project from its base into flat sheets or lamellae. Easier said than done!

Passing over some groups of animals with ciliary photoreceptors (see Eakin, 1972), I shall leap down the animal scale to the lowly jellyfish, which has a good contribution to make to this evolutionary story. My associates Jane Westfall and Jean Brandenburger and I have studied the eyecups (ocelli) of the beautiful hydromedusan *Polyorchis penicillatus* (Eakin and Westfall, 1962*b*; Eakin and Brandenburger, unpublished). The animal is bell-shaped, approx-imately 50 mm high and 30 mm in diameter, and fringed with as many as a hundred or more tentacles (Fig. 20). A bright, reddish purple eyecup, 180 μm in diameter, is situated on the outer surface and at the base of each tentacle. The eyecup consists of a single layer of cells of two types intermingling with each other—sensory and supportive cells (Fig. 21). The former bear the ciliary photo-receptors, the latter the pigment granules.

The sensory cilium of the hydromedusan is a long shaft with many cylindrical microvilli springing from its surface along its entire length (Figs. 22, 23). The villi are neither straight nor regularly arranged. They interdigitate with villous extensions from the adja-cent pigmented cells, filling the cavity of the eyecup with a tangle of processes, misidentified by earlier workers as a lens (Little, 1914) or a vitreous body (Linko, 1900). Cross sections of the cilia (Fig. 23) reveal a $9 \times 2 + 2$ pattern of microtubules! I speculate that at the coelenterate level of evolution of ciliary photoreceptors, the central microtubules, characteristic of all motile cilia, had not yet disappeared. Are the enzyme-containing arms present on the doub-

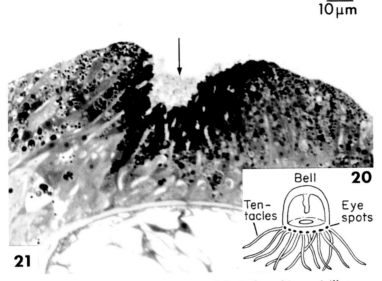

10 μm

Bell **20**

Ten-
tacles

Eye
spots

21

Fig. 20. Sketch of hydromedusan jellyfish, *Polyorchis penicillatus*.

Fig. 21. Light micrograph (hereafter abbreviated LM) of ocellus of *P. penicillatus* showing pigmented and sensory (white streaks) cells. Arrow indicates mass of processes from distal ends of sensory and pigmented cells. × 730. Heretofore unpublished, Eakin and Brandenburger.

lets? To answer this question Jean Brandenburger and I recently made a restudy of the eyecups of *Polyorchis*. Although there are some thin spokes (radial linkages, Warner, 1972) between the doublets and singlets, and strands (peripheral linkages) between the doublets, the arms were lacking. Moreover, the arrangement of the doublets differs from that of motile cilia in showing a greater variation in the distances between doublets and in the shape of the axoneme, which is frequently oval or irregular in cross-sectional outline.

One final step down is possible in this history of light-sensitive cilia—to the protista, the most primitive group of truly cellular organisms (eukaryotes), where plant and animal kingdoms merge. There are some protists (*Euglena gracilis*, for example) with eyespots in which the light-sensitive organelle is a motile cilium, only slightly modified. It has a swelling (paraflagellar body) at its base

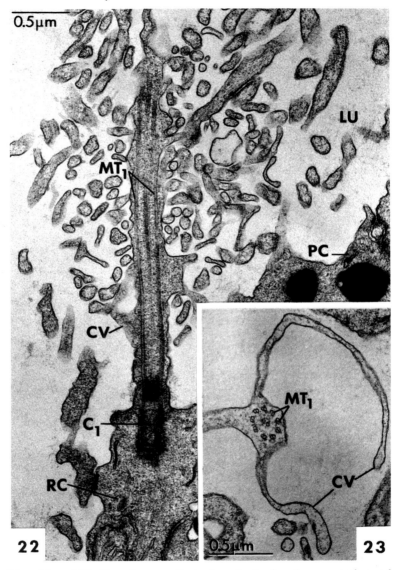

Figs. 22 and 23. Em of, respectively, longitudinal and cross sections of photoreceptor from ocellus of *P. penicillatus*. C_1, distal centriole (kinetosome); cv, microvilli from sensory cilium; lu, lumen of eyecup; MT_1, microtubules (axoneme) in cilium; pc, pigmented cell; rc, sensory cell. × 31,000 (Fig. 22); × 34,000 (Fig. 23). Eakin and Brandenburger, from Eakin (1970).

which is believed to contain the photopigment (see Grell, 1968). I regret that I am unable to illustrate this photoreceptor for lack of good electron micrographs. The ciliary swelling is shaded on one side by a cup-shaped layer (stigma) of red pigment. The rotational swimming movements of the organism cause an alternation of illumination and shadowing of the base of the cilium with laterally directed light. If the organism redirects the path of advancement toward the light, the receptor is continuously illuminated. Here, then, is the beginning of an eye, a structure to absorb radiant energy and transform it into chemical or electrical messages which inform the organism about the direction, intensity, and perhaps other qualities of the light reaching it. And it is instructive that nature used the cilium, already evolved for locomotion, as the organelle for photoreception.

Outmoded Thermostat

In tracing the history of the pineal foramen at the outset of this chapter I began with fossil reptiles possessing large foramina and went back in time to the beginnings of a photoreceptor. I return to my starting point to proceed forward in time toward reader and author, who lack third eyes. But why was the neat, beautiful parietal eye lost in the evolution of birds and mammals? Because the fossil record offers small assistance in answering this question, we are forced to rely more upon fancy than upon fact.

For what it is worth, let us briefly consider the ancient reptiles which were presumably the ancestors of mammals or their near relatives. They have been called mammal-like reptiles (therapsids). The distinction between a reptile and a mammal is one of definition and sometimes is not easily made. The zoologist defines a mammal as a vertebrate with mammary glands, hair, relatively constant bodily temperature (often less correctly referred to as warm-bloodedness), and a diaphragm, the muscular partition between thorax and abdomen used in breathing. These are features which are not preserved in the fossil record, as a rule, although bones may give hints regarding them. The paleontologist uses other criteria to separate reptiles and mammals, such as the nature of the connection between the lower jaw and the cranium. If mammae, hair, and diaphragm evolved before the mammalian jaw joint (dentary-squamosal)—and this is likely, according to A. S. Brink (1956) of South Africa—then perhaps the animals under consideration should be called reptile-like mammals instead of mammal-like reptiles.

My colleague Robert Stebbins has studied the pineal foramen of fossil reptiles that were on or near the line that presumably led to mammals. He has graciously allowed me to quote his findings and conclusions and to reproduce a few figures from his unpublished paper. Measurements by Stebbins show that the pineal foramen was large in some of the mammal-like reptiles, even larger than the foramen magnum. In several forms the foramen and the pineal canal through the cranial roof may have accommodated both a parietal eye and the epiphysis, the former being situated at the tip of the latter as in some modern lizards (for examples, a chameleon, *Chameleo*, and an alligator lizard, *Gerrhonotus*). In other species studied by Stebbins the pineal foramen was small, some having an area only 2 or 3 percent of that of the foramen magnum. In another line of mammal-like reptiles, the dog-tooth reptiles (cynodonts), Dr. Brink (1956) reports that the pineal foramen was either small or totally lacking. Although these reptiles are not believed to be the true ancestral stock of mammals, Brink presents evidence that they may have been "warm-blooded."

An example of the mammal-like reptiles studied by Stebbins is *Lystrosaurus murrayi*. He examined ten skulls of this species collected in South Africa (Triassic, Lystrosaurus Zone, Tweefontein, Middleburg, Cape Province). A specimen was sectioned mediallv (sagittally), and a latex impression was made of the cranial cavity (Fig. 24A). The pineal foramen was about one-third the area of the foramen magnum (4.5 $\times$ 4.0 mm and 13 $\times$ 7 mm, respectively) (see Fig. 24B). According to Stebbins: "The pineal opening in *Lystrosaurus murrayi* may have been situated above or only slightly anterior to the epiphysis, and the parietal eye and epiphysis may have been closely associated if not actually in contact. If the skull is held with the eyes and nasal openings on a horizontal line, in keeping with the animal's presumed amphibious habits, the pineal axis, as estimated, is directed upwards" (see Fig. 24C).

Now, thermal regulation in mammals and birds involves internal

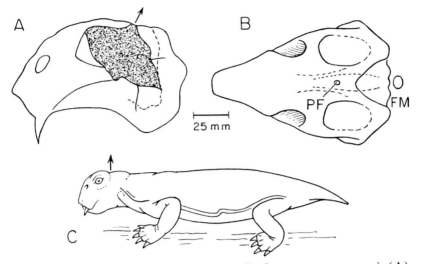

Fig. 24. South African mammal-like reptile *Lystrosaurus murrayi*. (A) Longitudinal section of head showing brain cavity (stippled) and direction of pineal canal (arrow). (B) Top of skull showing parietal or pineal foramen (PF); oval (FM) beside skull represents size of foramen magnum. (C) Reconstruction of animal by artist (Stebbins); arrow indicates visual axis of third eye. From unpublished paper by Robert C. Stebbins; Emily E. Reid, delineator.

mechanisms for controlling both the production and the conservation of heat and, conversely, its reduction and dissipation, depending upon the external temperature. Reptiles, on the other hand, rely upon solar radiation as their principal source of heat, and they regulate their bodily temperature by moving between sunlight and shade as needed. In Chapter 5 I shall discuss the theory, which Stebbins and I advanced (Stebbins and Eakin, 1958), that the reptilian parietal eye participates in this thermal regulation by serving as a dosimeter of solar radiation. If this thesis is correct, then the evolution of the mammalian and avian mechanisms of thermal adjustment rendered the third eye obsolete. There was no longer any tendency for natural selection, in the Darwinian sense, to preserve the eye, much less to improve it. Stebbins further speculates that a reduction in the size of the pineal foramen and lateral compression of the pineal canal may be correlated with the enlargement of the jaw muscles associated with carnivorous habits. So, to state the fate of the third eye teleologically, since it was no longer needed as a dosimeter of solar radiation, the hole that it had occupied was filled with bone to increase the strength of the skull. The eye had to go.

But the Epiphysis Survived

The epiphysis, or pineal body, has already been mentioned in the introduction of our third character, the lamprey, in connection with its upper median eye. The epiphysis varies from an oval vesicle on the roof of the brain in lower vertebrates to a conical body deeply recessed between lobes of the brain in higher vertebrates. The Greeks, Romans, and early French writers knew the structure, and, being impressed with its resemblance in higher vertebrates to a pine cone, they gave it the name of conical body (Greek, *konos*, 'cone'; *soma*, 'body') or pineal body (Latin, *pineale*, 'pine cone'; *corpus*, 'body'). The term *epiphysis*, a synonym for *pineal body*, comes from two Greek words, *epi*, meaning 'upon,' and *phyesthai*, 'to grow,' in reference to the dorsal outgrowth of the epiphysis from the embryonic brain (see Chapter 4).

Now, the epiphysis also possesses ciliary photoreceptors that are similar to those in median eyes. There appears to be a trend toward degeneration in the epiphysial receptors, however, as one proceeds from cyclostomes to mammals. This story is beautifully presented in an impressive monograph recently published by Jean-Pierre Collin (1969*b*). The epiphysis declined in photoreceptoral function until there were only a few rudimentary receptors in some birds and none in mammals. Meanwhile the secretory activity of the organ increased to the point where in most birds and in all mammals this appears to be its only function. Correlated with these changes in the nature of the chief cells of the organ, Collin points out that there were alterations also in the neural pathways—namely, the disappearance above the amphibia of certain cells (ganglion) specialized for receiving and transmitting nervous messages originating in the photoreceptoral cells and the absence thereafter of a type of neural junction (those with synaptic ribbons) which are highly characteristic of photosensory organs. Finally, efforts to record electrical responses to light from avian pineals have so far been unsuccessful (Morita, 1966*b*; Ralph and Dawson, 1968). Continuous spontaneous activity has been demonstrated in mammalian epiphyses by several investigators. Some (Taylor and Wilson, 1970) found that the electrical activity in a rat pineal body was inhibited by illumination of the animal (lateral eyes intact). The inhibition was stated to be mediated by the retina of the lateral eye. The use of certain neural blocking reagents suggested, moreover, that the pathway to the pineal body is the autonomic nervous system (postganglionic sympathetic fibers from the superior cervical ganglion). Other workers recorded spontaneous electrical activity from a rat epiphysis which was dependent, in part, upon influences from the lateral eyes. I know of no observation of neural activity resulting from direct illumination of a mammalian epiphysis separated from the rest of the body. Biochemical changes in avian pineal organs do occur with daily illumination, but these are believed to be mediated by neural pathways between lateral eyes and epiphyses (Quay, 1972).* Further research is needed on the neurophysiology of avian and mammalian pineal organs.

* The structure and function of the epiphysis lies beyond the scope of this work. The reader is referred, therefore, to the following treatises: Tilney and Warren (1919); Gladstone and Wakeley (1940); Kitay and Altschule (1954); Thiéblot and Le Bars (1955); Kappers and Schadé, eds. (1965); Wurtman, Axelrod, and Kelly (1968); Ralph (1970); a symposium on the pineal organized by Reiter (1970); Wolstenholme and Knight, eds. (1971); and Quay (1973).

3
Structure

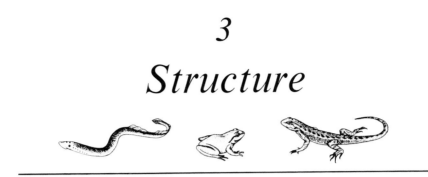

Our characters have been introduced, and the evolutionary history of the third eye and of ciliary photoreceptors has been sketched. Before the function of the eye can be properly discussed, however, a more detailed account of its structure is necessary. I admonish my students that if they cannot be excited by anatomy for its own sake, as their instructor is, they should learn it for a full understanding of physiology.

Reptilian Third Eye

A CENTURY OF STUDY.

It was a hundred years ago that the third eye of lizards was first noted by a German biologist, Franz Leydig, professor of zoology and comparative anatomy at Tübingen University. He is better known for his description of the male-hormone-secreting cells of the testis (called Leydig's cells or interstitial cells). Leydig (1872) studied several European lizards (three species of *Lacerta* and the Slow Worm *Anguis fragilis*) and found a small, round, pigmented organ on the top of the embryonic brain and under the large median dorsal scale of the adult brain. He characterized the cells composing the body as long and cylindrical, arranged to form a shallow, upwardly directed cup. Its wall possessed a black, pigmented band, which feature made it visible to the unaided eye. Leydig called the structure a frontal organ (*Stirnorgan*), and he suggested that it might be glandular in function.

It was fourteen years later (1886) before the eyelike nature of Leydig's organ, which designation was used by earlier workers, was determined by Henri W. de Graaf of Leiden, who described the retina and lens and even anticipated the discovery of the light-sensitive elements of the eye by his statement that the layer on the inner surface of the organ reminded him of the layer of rods of a retina. He gave a diagrammatic sketch of the eye which is quite accurate. Very shortly thereafter in the same year W. Baldwin Spencer (1886*a*), then an assistant and fellow of Lincoln College, Oxford University, published the first account of the third eye in the New Zealand reptile (*Hatteria punctatus* = *Sphenodon punctatus*) that I mentioned in Chapter 1. This is not a lizard, although lizardlike in form; it belongs to another subdivision (order) of the class Reptilia—namely, the Rhynchocephalia. Spencer (1886*b*) also produced a long paper on the presence and structure of the parietal eye in twenty-eight species of lizards plus *Sphenodon*. The work was the most complete account of the organ to date, and it was well illustrated.

In 1905 the Czech F. K. Studnička of Brünn (Gregor Mendel's home town) published a book entitled *Die Parietalorgane*, which summarized the early literature on the pineal-parietal complex of all classes of vertebrates from cyclostomes to mammals, to which he added much new information from his own studies. He remarked that the investigations of these organs had become so numerous in the twenty-five years prior to his work that he had had to survey a literature of almost three hundred titles. Imagine my task after another seventy-five years! In comparison to Studnička's review, mine is sketchy indeed. His book was abundantly illustrated, and one set of his diagrams showing the comparative anatomy of the pineal-parietal complex in vertebrates has been frequently reproduced, even in recent times. In fact, I considered including it here.

In 1910 two monographic studies on reptilian third eyes were produced. The Russian M. Nowikoff, a comparative anatomist at the University of Moscow, published a magnificent work on the structure, development, and function of the parietal eye in several species of European lizards. It was written in simple German, to my great delight when I was a struggling beginner in that language. The figures were meticulously and beautifully delineated and lithographed. The same should be said, incidentally, of the works of Leydig and Spencer. I never cease to marvel over the perspicacity of the biologists of that period (from about 1880 to 1920) when the great studies in microscopic anatomy were conducted. They pushed the light microscope to its limits and even foreshadowed discoveries made later with the electron microscope. The second work completed in 1910 (actually published in early 1911) was that of Arthur Dendy, professor of zoology at King's College, University of London, on the structure and development of the pineal organs in the New Zealand tuatara. He greatly extended the frontier of knowledge of the third eye in this unique reptile, beyond that provided by the earlier investigation of Spencer.

Research on third eyes of lizards was limited after 1911 until the late 1950s, when there was a remarkable recrudescence of interest in the subject. The new anatomical studies, which made use of electron microscopy and staining procedures to identify specific substances (histochemistry), provided the basis of the following account of the structure of the reptilian parietal eye. Incidentally, not all reptiles possess the parietal eye, as Spencer (1886*b*) first discovered. It is lacking in turtles, snakes, alligators and their relatives, and in several families of lizards, such as the whiptails (Teiidae), geckos (Gekkonidae), and beaded lizards (Helodermatidae).

GENERAL MORPHOLOGY.

The relationship of the third eye of a lizard to its brain is shown in a median section through the head (Fig. 25) of an adult blue-belly. The microscopic preparation figured here was skillfully made by Dr. Robert Ortman for Dr. Stebbins and me many years ago. The parietal eye (PA) lies above the cerebrum (CM), the large anterior division of the brain, and in the pineal foramen (PF) of the cranium, the history of which we traced in Chapter 2. The reader should be reminded of the small size of the parietal eye (about 0.2 mm in diameter). The large, clear space beneath the eye and roof of the cranium is due to shrinkage of the brain by the preservative (fix-

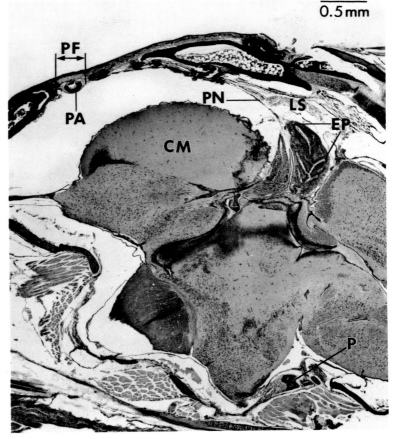

Fig. 25. Lm of median longitudinal (sagittal) section of head of *S. occidentalis*. cm, cerebrum of brain; ep, epiphysis; ls, large blood vessel (longitudinal sinus); p, pituitary gland; pa, parietal eye; pf, parietal foramen; pn, parietal nerve. × 24. Stebbins, Eakin, and Ortman, from Stebbins and Eakin (1958).

ative). Behind the cerebrum lie several organs, such as the epiphysis (ep) which I mentioned already as being outside the scope of this work, although it is closely associated with the parietal eye developmentally and functionally. Parietal eye and epiphysis are also connected anatomically, by the parietal nerve, a segment of which (pn) is to be observed in this section.

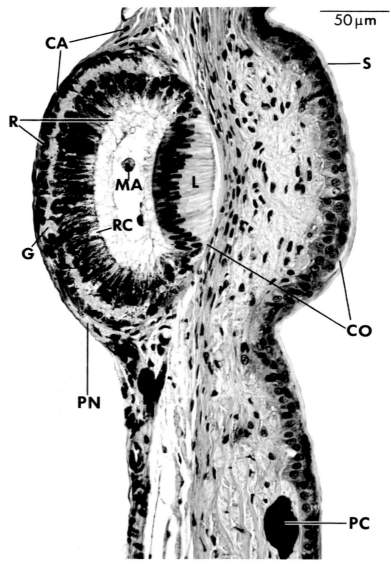

Fig. 26. Lм of median longitudinal (sagittal) section of parietal eye of *S. occidentalis*. CA, capsule; CO, cornea; G, ganglion cell; L, lens; MA, macrophage; PC, pigmented cell; PN, parietal nerve; R, retina; RC, receptor cell; S, scale. × 360. Heretofore unpublished, Eakin and Ferlatte.

At higher magnification (Fig. 26) one sees the structures already noted in the introduction: cornea (co), lens (l), and retina (r). The cornea is composed of an inner, highly fibrous layer; a middle, less dense stratum, which is continuous with the dermis of the skin; and an outer epidermal layer. The latter contributes by secretion to the large scale (interparietal) above the eye (see Fig. 1). The cornea is fused with the lens, a palisade of elongate, cylindrical cells whose nuclei lie at their basal ends. (The slit between cornea and lens in the figure is an artifact.) A fibrous capsule (ca) encloses the eye and attaches it to the skin. The parietal nerve (pa) leaves the retina, as I shall detail later, passes through the capsule, and courses posteriorly under the roof of the cranium and then ventrally to the epiphysis and the brain.

RETINAL COMPONENTS.

There are three kinds of cells in the retina: sensory, supportive, and ganglion. The sensory cells (rc, Fig. 26) are columnar units devoid of black pigment, which bear receptoral processes, one per cell, at their upper (distal) ends. The processes cannot be clearly seen in Figure 26; they lie in the mesh of coagulated fluid (humor) in the cavity (lumen) of the eye. The reader will note that the forward projection of the processes into the cavity of the eye is unlike the position of rods and cones in the lateral eyes of vertebrates. The latter extend backwards from the retina and the incoming light; this position is said to be inverse, whereas that of the third eye processes is designated converse. The explanation of the difference in orientation of the receptoral elements in median and lateral eyes is to be found in their development (see Chapter 4). The nuclei of the sensory cells form a band near the middle of the retina, largely obscured by the pigment in the supportive cells.

The supportive cells are also columnar units interspersed among the sensory cells. The abundant pigment granules, presumably composed of melanin, are concentrated in the distal halves of the supportive cells. The pigment is movable, as demonstrated by Nowikoff (1910) in experiments on European lizards (*Lacerta agilis* and *Anguis fragilis*). It moves distally in light-adapted animals and basally in animals placed in total darkness. I confirmed this observation by similar experiments on *S. occidentalis* and *Uta stansburiana*. The nuclei of the supportive cells lie peripherally, just inside the capsule of the eye, together with some pigment granules.

Ganglion cells are much fewer than the other retinal elements. They are identified by their large size, large nuclei, and basal position in the nonpigmented band of the retina. One ganglion cell is indicated (G) in Figure 26.

Outer Segment of Receptoral Process.

Electron microscopy has enabled us to add much detail to the anatomical picture just given. An electron micrograph of a sensory process in the third eye of a fence lizard was shown earlier in Figure 9. The distal or outer segment (os) is, as we learned in Chapter 1, a modified cilium. It consists of a stack of disks or flattened sacs which are open to the cavity of the eye, attesting to their origin by outfolding of the membrane of the cilium. The evenly spaced disks measure about 2.5 μm in diameter and 250–300 A in thickness.*

Upper and lower membranes of a disk are comparable in thickness to that of cell membranes (about 75 A), and the space within a disk (intradiskal space) measures 100–150 A in width. As the space between disks (interdiskal) has roughly the same width, the repeat distance is approximately 400 A. Thus, there are around 25 disks per micrometer of sensory process. I have found some outer segments in the third eye of *Sceloporus* to be at least 10 μm in length. Accordingly, an individual outer segment may contain 250 or more disks. The French investigator André Petit (1968) reports that the processes in the third eye of a European lizard, *Anguis fragilis*, measure from 10 to 17 μm and have from 250 to 435 disks. Although these estimates of the number of sensory units seem large, it has been

---

* Formerly, the millionth part of a meter was called a micron, symbolized by μ and the billionth part of a meter was termed a millimicron (mμ). Nowadays, the former is frequently designated a micrometer (μm), the latter a nanometer (nm). And the commonly used linear measure in ultrastructural studies is the angstrom unit (A), which is one tenth of a nanometer or 10^{-10} meters. Fashions in terminology change, although not so frequently, fortunately, as those of dress. The next change will probably be a replacement of the angstrom unit (named for the Swedish physicist Anders Jöns Ångström, 1814–1874) because of the trend to abandon terms bearing the names of scientists. A logical designation would be *desinanometer*. But, must our scientific language lose all its color and historical associations with persons?

calculated that there are close to 2,000 disks in certain rods (so-called red rods) of a frog (Nilsson, 1965).

One might ask what holds the disks together. They are indeed fragile, and rough treatment, mechanical or chemical, can cause them to separate or swell or shrink. (Incidentally, these artifacts resulting from preparation for electron microscopy make it difficult to give exact measurements of the disks.) But I have not answered the question. The disks are held together by the shaft of the outer segment (the cilium). Each disk is open to the lumen of the eye, the consequence of its mode of formation: by foldings of the ciliary membrane. But the invaginations do not cut completely through the cilium. The uncut side is a shaft to which the disks are attached. The picture is like a loaf of French bread that is incompletely sliced. The slices are like the disks, and the part of the loaf to which the slices are connected resembles the shaft of the outer segment. The dough is the counterpart of the cytoplasm. The simile breaks down, however, when, one looks at the individual slices of bread—their cut surfaces are not covered with crust! Another third eye process (shown in Fig. 27) was cut in a plane which did not pass through the shaft. Consequently, the disks appear to be unconnected, like a pile of coins (Fig. 28). Had the section been taken in a plane at right angles to this one (along the arrows on the outer segment, Fig. 27), the picture would have been like that in Figure 9.

Embedded within the cytoplasm of the shaft of the outer segment (cilium) is the remarkable bundle (axoneme) of microtubules mentioned in Chapter 1. These stiffeners, one of which (MT_1) may be well seen in Figures 9 and 27, extend up from the base of the shaft for a considerable distance, maybe half the length of the process. Below the first disk the outer segment narrows to a slender neck, called a connecting piece (CP), that attaches the outer segment to that part of the process termed the inner segment (IS). The microtubules pass through the connecting piece and into the inner segment as far as a small cylindrical structure (C_1), variously known as distal centriole, axial centriole, basal body, and kinetosome. Biologists love words! If one examines a cross section of the connecting piece (Fig. 10), one sees that the microtubules are arranged in the now-familiar ring of nine doublets; central microtubules are absent. The ciliary nature of the sensory processes of pineal eyes was first estab-

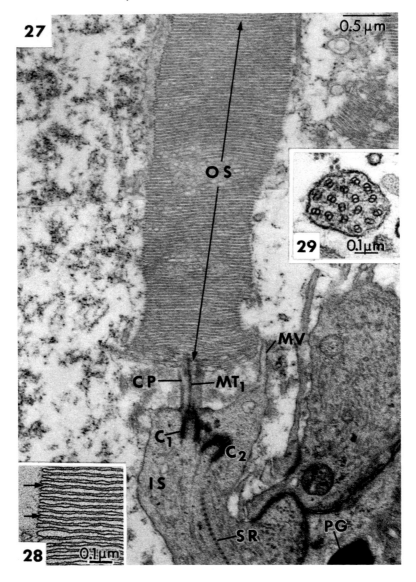

lished by Dr. Jane Westfall and me on *S. occidentalis* (Eakin and Westfall, 1959, 1960) and by Willem Steyn (1959*a*, 1960) in South Africa on the lizard *Cordylus polyzonus*. It is only fair to say, how-however, that the early light microscopists were close to the truth. Nowikoff (1910), for example, thought that the processes projecting into the lumen of the eye were fused cilia.

Mistakes in development (anomalies) are sometimes interesting, instructive, even humorous to the embryologist, if they do not seriously interfere with normal function. Exceptions to the usual pattern of nine doublets of microtubules in cilia are well known. Figure 29 illustrates an abnormal axoneme which Millie Miller Ferlatte recently found in a parietal eye of a *Sceloporus* embryo. It has sixteen doublets irregularly arranged in the ciliary shaft. Something went awry in the formation of microtubules in this cilium. Nature simply overproduced.

Inner Segment of Receptoral Process.

The inner segment is actually the distal part of the receptor cell, which extends into the lumen of the eye beyond the level of cell-to-cell attachments. Light microscopists formerly stated that inner segments of retinal processes projected through lacunae in a limiting membrane (Walls, 1942). Electron microscopy, however, reveals no limiting membrane on the surface of a retina. The light microscopist was observing the line of cell contacts, which are bands of close apposition of neighboring cells. The most prominent component of the junctional complexes are termed desmosomes, which

---

Fig. 27. EM of longitudinal section of photoreceptoral process in parietal eye of *S. occidentalis*. c_1, distal centriole (kinetosome); c_2, proximal or accessory centriole; CP, connecting piece; IS, inner segment of receptoral process; MT_1, microtubule in cilium; MV, microvillus; OS, outer segment of receptoral process; PG, pigment granule in supportive cell; SR, striated rootlet. Arrows indicate plane of section shown in Fig. 9. × 23,000. Heretofore unpublished, Eakin and Brandenburger.

Fig. 28. Enlargement of outer edges of disks shown in Fig. 27. Arrows indicate patency of disks. × 57,000. Heretofore unpublished, Eakin and Brandenburger.

Fig. 29. Abnormal connecting piece of photoreceptoral process from third eye of *S. occidentalis*. Instead of a ring of nine doublets, as seen in cross section, there are sixteen doublets. × 58,000. Heretofore unpublished, Eakin, Brandenburger, and Ferlatte.

bind the receptor cells to adjacent pigmented supportive cells (see below) somewhat as spot weldings hold pieces of metal together.

One of the major constituents of the inner segment is the centriolar apparatus. I have already described one element, the distal centriole, or kinetosome, from which the axoneme arises. Additionally, there is a second centriole adjacent and at right angles to the kinetosome. Both centrioles are bundles of nine triplets of microtubules (see Fig. 11). Leading down into the cell from the centrioles is a long, striated rootlet (sr, Figs. 9, 27). Alternating light bands (about 550 A wide) and dark bands (about 350 A wide) give the rootlet its striated appearance. One of the functions of the distal centriole is known; it is the organizer of the developing sensory process (see Chapter 4). The role of the accessory centriole, however, is enigmatic. The striated rootlet probably serves as an anchor for centrioles and axoneme, and not as a conductor of an excitation, as once thought.

The region around and below the centrioles has been called the ellipsoid by light microscopists. The term was chosen because this area in cone cells of a frog's lateral eye had that geometric shape. Ellipsoids stain heavily with fuchsin dye and were thought to be light-concentrating devices (Walls, 1942; Winston and Enoch, 1971). Electron microscopy of rod and cone ellipsoids has revealed a remarkable aggregation of mitochondria, small rodlets of varying size, which are exceedingly important in making energy available for a multitude of chemical reactions in cells, including those concerned with vision. The receptor cells of third eyes likewise possesses masses of mitochondria in their inner segments. They are particularly well shown in an amphibian third-eye receptor (m, Fig. 44) soon to be described. In the parietal eyes of *Sceloporus* and other lizards, however, mitochondria are not numerous in the upper end of the inner segment, but they are abundant farther down in the cell (not shown). Now that electron microscopy has demonstrated that the ellipsoid is an accumulation of mitochondria, I believe that the term should be discontinued. Morever, in the instance of a third eye, an example of a converse retina, the inner segment could not usefully serve as a light-guiding structure because the light first strikes the sensory processes.

Recent studies, such as those of my colleague on our Los Angeles campus Professor Richard Young (1970), have shown that in the lateral eye proteins are channeled from synthetic centers deep in the cell into the connecting piece, probably by the longitudinally oriented mitochondria and cytoplasmic microtubules in the inner segment. The technique used by Young and others is called autoradiography (self-radioactive–writing). Amino acids, the building blocks of proteins, are tagged with some radioactive element and administered to animals. After the amino acids have been distributed by the circulatory system to all parts of the body, the eyes are removed at varying times from different animals and are prepared for microscopy. Sections through the eyes are first coated with photographic emulsion in a darkroom under a faint red light and then are stored in total darkness for a few weeks. The emulsion is developed. A silver grain will appear in the emulsion, superimposed over the tissue, wherever there is a protein molecule containing the radioactive amino acid. By this procedure an investigator can plot the movement of proteins in a cell, such as a rod or a cone cell. From the connecting piece the proteins, and other metabolites as well, pass along the shaft of the outer segment, guided, perhaps, by the microtubules of the axoneme, and into the thin layers of cytoplasm between the disks. One protein in this stream is opsin, the major structural molecule of the disks. Moreover, opsin combined with retinaldehyde (a vitamin A derivative) becomes a photopigment, such as rhodopsin. At the moment we have no information on the specific photopigment of a parietal eye.

We know that the parietal eye is functional, however, because there are changes in electrical activity, which can be recorded from the retina (ERG) or parietal eye nerve when light to the eye is turned on or off. Moreover, I demonstrated (Eakin, 1964*b*) before the neuroelectrical recordings were made—although the paper was published afterwards—that a deficiency of vitamin A causes a breakdown in the outer segments of third-eye receptors in *S. occidentalis.* A fuller treatment of the evidence of function will be presented in Chapter 5. For the moment, let it be said that the eye contains a light-sensitive substance (or perhaps two or more substances, since it reacts differently to short and long wavelengths of light).

And we must assume that inner segments are involved in the transmission of excitations generated in the outer segments, on the basis of the neurophysiological studies and by analogy with the function of rods and cones in the lateral eyes of vertebrates. The impulses are presumed to be carried by the plasma membrane. Although delicate fingerlike extensions of the inner segment (MV, Fig. 27) embrace the outer segment, their functional role is not known. Professor George Wald, who has been a source of assistance and inspiration to me for many years, once proposed that similar villi surrounding the rods and cones of certain vertebrates (for examples, amphibians, monkey) be designated dendrites, although without implying that they are involved in the transmission of excitations (Wald, Brown, and Gibbons, 1963). To me, however, the use of *dendrite* does indeed imply a neural function—specifically, the generation of a neural response. It seems unlikely that any impulse generated in the outer segment would jump the extracellular space separating the outer segment and the villi unless their membranes were in intimate contact with each other. Such cell contacts have not been observed in either median or lateral eyes.

Body of Receptor Cell.

Moving basally in the sensory cell we come next to a region above the nucleus which the light microscopist has designated the paraboloid. Walls (1942) characterized paraboloids of retinal receptors in general as bodies which usually resist staining and which keep their paraboloid shape when expressed from living cells. He added that a paraboloid may have some important function other than its optical one. I believe that this term should also be discarded because the region so designated does not have a regular shape, and it does not serve an obvious optical function, especially in eyes with a converse retina. Moreover, electron microscopy now permits an ultrastructural characterization of this supranuclear region. It is a body of cisternae and granules.

For the reader unacquainted with the microscopist's jargon, cisternae are fluid-filled spaces, in the present instance belonging to an extensive network of channels, known as endoplasmic reticulum, which ramifies throughout a cell. The term is taken from the Latin *cisterna*, meaning 'reservoir.' The cisternae in the supranuclear area of a parietal eye receptor vary from irregular, interconnected spaces (Fig. 30) to organized stacks of more or less parallel cister-

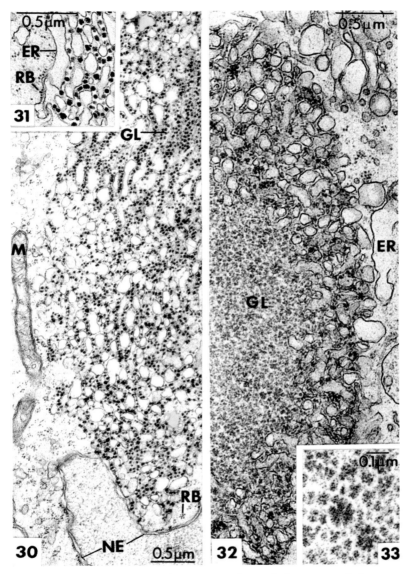

Figs. 30–33. EM of supranuclear aggregations of cisternae and glycogen (so-called paraboloid) in sensory cells of parietal eye of *S. occidentalis*. ER, cisternae of endoplasmic reticulum; GL, glycogen granules (beta particles in Figs. 30 and 31, alpha particles in Figs. 32 and 33); M, mitochondrion; NE, nuclear envelope; RB, ribosomes. × 23,000 (Fig. 30); × 31,000 (Figs. 31, 32); × 62,000 (Fig. 33). Eakin and Westfall, from Eakin (1964*b*).

nae, as shown by Petit (1968). The membranous walls of the cisternae are smooth—that is, devoid of attached small granules (ribosomes). These smooth cisternae of endoplasmic reticulum, however, connect with the granular ER. In Figure 31 one sees the continuity between granular and smooth ER. Note the small size (about 150 A) of the ribosomes (RB) which cling also to the outer membrane of the nuclear envelope (NE, Fig. 30) and which occur as free ribosomes (that is, unattached to membranes) in the cytoplasm. Can I assume that the reader knows the function of ribosomes? They are sites of synthesis of proteins, hence indispensable cell structures.

The larger, black granules in Figures 30 and 31 are not ribosomes but deposits of glycogen. The size of the individual granule is in the order of several hundred or a thousand angstrom units, and although they are associated with ER membranes they are unattached. Most glycogen granules are clusters of subunits, called beta particles. The clusters, designated alpha particles, are often starlike figures (Figs. 32, 33) and are so concentrated in the center of the supranuclear region that cisternae are excluded. The glycogen nature of these granules is suggested by their digestibility with the glycogen-splitting enzyme alpha amylase, and their positive staining with a histochemical procedure, the PAS reaction, which colors red certain carbohydrates, including glycogen (Eakin, Quay, and Westfall, 1961; Petit, 1968).

The considerable variation in the appearance of the glycogen deposits I attributed tentatively to seasonal differences (Eakin, 1964*a*). Petit (1968) reported that lizards (*Anguis fragilis*) subjected to several days of illumination exhibited an increase in glycogen granules and a reduction in the membranous components of their "paraboloids." This observation does not agree, however, with our impression (Eakin, Quay and Westfall, 1961) that glycogen is more abundant in the third eyes of dark-adapted *S. occidentalis* than in parietal eyes of light-adapted lizards. Petit (1968) postulated that there are successive phases in the development of a "paraboloid," the first one being similar to the appearance in Figure 30, the final one like that in Figure 32. More work on this important region of the receptor cell is needed.

Receptor Cell Axon.

In our journey down the receptor cell we come next to its nucleus. But there is nothing unique about this all-important structure, so I pass on to the basal end of the cell, which narrows to form a nerve fiber called a neurite or axon. To the best of our knowledge, it is relatively short, as nerve fibers go, extending only a few micrometers to make contact with a second retinal element, the ganglion cell. I qualified this statement because the axons are difficult to follow in ultrathin sections since they are not straight. Rarely can one follow an axon for more than a segment of its length unless special efforts are made, such as preparing a long uninterrupted series of sections for careful, tedious tracing of a given axon. It is possible, although unlikely, that some axons of the sensory cells bypass the ganglion cells and enter directly into the parietal nerve.

Each axon terminal (T, Fig. 34) contains mitochondria (M), stacks or whorls of cisternae with glycogen granules (Fig. 35) resembling those in the supranuclear center discussed above, longitudinally ordered microtubules (MT), and vesicles (SV). The vesicles are uniform in size (about 300 A, according to my measurement; 440–550 A in *Anguis fragilis,* according to Petit, 1968) and relatively electron-lucent. At certain places on the surface of the terminal the vesicles are aggregated and the cell membrane is thickened. These regions are called synapses; here nervous impulses are transferred from the terminals of the receptor cells to ganglion cells. Accordingly, the vesicles are termed synaptic vesicles. There is evidence, which will not be reviewed here, that the passage of nervous impulses from receptor to ganglion cells depends upon the release of substances within the synaptic vesicles.

An additional feature of a synapse between a terminal of a receptor cell and a process (dendrite) of a ganglion cell is a dense bar, called a synaptic ribbon (SNR, Fig. 34), which is usually oriented perpendicularly to the membrane of the receptor terminal and surrounded by synaptic vesicles. Figure 34 shows two terminals (T) of sensory cells in synaptic contact with a dendrite (GD) of a ganglion cell. Note the difference in density of cytoplasm between the two nerve fibers. The membranes of the receptor terminals immediately below the synaptic ribbons show unusual, small, globular bodies.

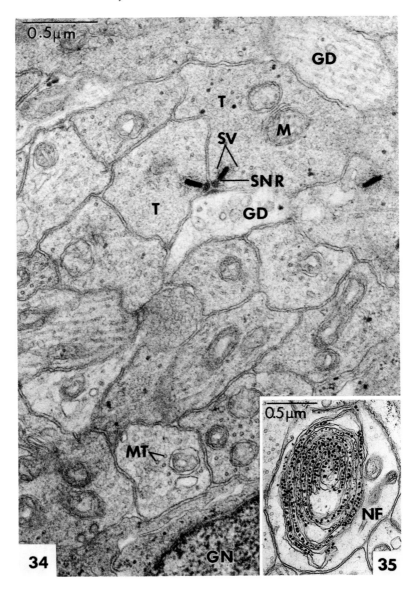

Each density and its associated synaptic ribbon look like an exclamation point! Since nervous impulses pass from terminal to dendrite, these dense structures are said to be presynaptic. The adjacent membrane (postsynaptic) of the dendrite is also thickened by some kind of deposit on the cytoplasmic side. Pre- and postsynaptic membranes are separated by a space, the synaptic cleft. In the present instance two receptor cells share a common postsynaptic site. The advantage of such an arrangement will be considered in Chapter 5.

Rod Versus Cone.

Before continuing an account of the structure of the retina of the third eye of *Sceloporus*, I should remark on the kind of sensory cell just described. Is it like a rod or a cone, the principal categories of receptors in the retinas of lateral eyes? When I first reflected on this question, I concluded that it was conelike, for a couple of reasons. Every disk was open to the lumen of the eye along its rim, as shown in the accompanying diagram (Fig. 36). As noted earlier, this feature is characteristic of nonmammalian cones. Second, a supranuclear body of glycogen granules and cisternae is more frequently found in cones than in rods. I was surprised to learn, however, that the parietal-eye receptor of *Sceloporus* lacked an oil droplet, whereas the cones in the lateral eye of this lizard have large droplets of lipid, one per cell embedded in the mass of mitochondria of the inner segment. But there are oil droplets in the inner segments of the third-eye receptors of the Granite Night Lizard *Xantusia henshawi* (see Eakin and Westfall, 1960). Moreover, Petit (1968) reports droplets of lipids in the inner segments of third-eye receptors in the limbless lizard *Anguis fragilis*.

A feature which clearly distinguishes rods and cones in certain

---

Fig. 34. EM of nerve fibers (neuropile) in retina of third eye of *S. occidentalis*. GD, dendrites of ganglion cells; GN, nucleus of ganglion cell; M, mitochondrion; MT, microtubules (neurotubules); SNR, synaptic ribbon; SV, synaptic vesicles; T, terminals of sensory cell axons. × 40,000. Heretofore unpublished, Eakin and Brandenburger.

Fig. 35. EM of cross section of a nerve fiber (NF) in retina of third eye of *S. occidentalis*, showing whorl of membranes enclosing granules of glycogen. × 26,000. Eakin and Westfall, from Eakin (1964*b*).

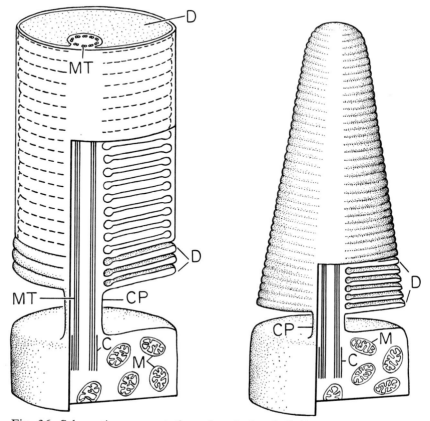

Fig. 36. Schematic representation of typical rod (left) and typical cone (right) from lateral eyes of lower vertebrates. C, centriole; CP, connecting piece; D, disks; M, mitochondria; MT, microtubules (axoneme). Modified from Young (1970); Emily E. Reid, delineator.

amphibians and mammals (for example, monkey) is the pattern of growth: continuous in the former, discontinuous after maturation in the latter (Young, 1971*a*, 1971*b*). Electron microscopy has shown that the tips of rods, involving blocks of disks, are periodically shed and incorporated into the adjacent cells of the pigmented epithelium, where they are broken down. New disks are continually added to the base of the outer segment by invaginations of the ciliary membrane (do not forget that the outer segment is a cilium). Young (see 1971*b*) has proved the correctness of this interpretation of the microscopist by experiments demonstrating the incorporation of radioactive amino acids into the proteins in the basalmost disks of a rod. With time this labeled group of disks moved distally, eventually became detached and engulfed by the pigmented epithelial cells in much the same manner as an amoeba or a white blood cell incorporates (phagocytizes), respectively, a food organism or a bacterium which has gained entry into the body. A rod practices recycling in an exemplary way.

But not cones. There is no evidence from either anatomical studies or the experiments of Young that cones continue production of new disks after full growth has been reached, unless there is a loss of the outer segment, in which event a new one is formed. Autoradiography of incorporated amino acids showed only weak, diffuse distribution of new protein in the outer segments of cones. What is the growth pattern of parietal-eye receptors? Is it rodlike or conelike? One does not regularly see many sloughed tips of outer segments in the parietal eyes of lizards, although they are abundant in the third eyes of frogs and lampreys. It is probable that any disks shed are phagocytized by large amoebalike cells, called macrophages, which wander in the lumen of the eye (Eakin, Quay, and Westfall, 1961; Petit, 1968). Petit (1968) has observed stacks of lamellae within the macrophages, strong evidence of engulfment of exfoliated disks. In this respect the macrophages perform the same function as the pigmented epithelium of the retina in the lateral eye. A macrophage (MA) in a third eye of *Sceloporus* may be seen in Figure 26.

As yet no autoradiography has been conducted on a parietal eye, but Bunt and Kelly (1971) have made chemical and autoradiographic studies on the epiphysis of a frog, *Rana pipiens*. As indicated earlier, epiphyses of many vertebrates below birds and mammals contain photoreceptors similar to those in third eyes. Therefore, the findings of Bunt and Kelly are pertinent to this discussion of parietal-eye receptors in *Sceloporus*. These investigators found that the pattern of distribution of new (radioactive) protein was similar to that observed in cones by Young—namely, diffuse over the outer segment instead of in a discrete band of disks, as in rods. Bunt and Kelly also reported radioactivity in macrophages in the lumen of the organ. Moreover, these cells contain stacks of membranes resembling outer segments and a digestive enzyme (acid phosphatase) which would assist in the destruction of the engulfed material. These last observations suggest a turnover in the outer segments of the frog epiphysis, a rod feature!

Jean Brandenburger and I discovered a histochemical difference between rods and cones in the lateral eyes of two species of frogs (Eakin and Brandenburger, 1970). This is the degree of stainability of the cytoplasm of the outer segments by prolonged action of unbuffered osmium tetroxide at 40°C. The rod cytoplasm is heavily stained, whereas that of cones contains only a light sprinkling of granules of osmium black, the precipitate resulting from a change (reduction) in the osmium tetroxide by compounds in the cytoplasm. We have applied this technique of osmium impregnation to the third eye of *Sceloporus* (heretofore unpublished) in the hope of throwing some light on the classification of third-eye receptors. The outer segments were blackened (Fig. 37) like the rods of the amphibian lateral eye. Moreover, Ueck (1971) obtained a similar result in the epiphysial photoreceptors of a frog, *Rana pipiens*. For what it is worth, this line of evidence suggests that the parietal-eye receptors are rodlike in the availability of free reactants with osmium tetroxide.

Another difference between rods and cones of lateral retinas lies in the greater susceptibility to fixation artifact of cones than rods. I refer to a breakdown of disks into vesicles by short fixation with osmium tetroxide that is often shown by cones but not by rods (Eakin, 1965). The disks in the outer segments of median-eye receptors have this same tendency to vesiculate when poorly fixed with osmium tetroxide (see Fig. 37). The basis for the fragility of cones is not clear. I have suggested that it is due, at least in part, to the lack of the sturdy rims which rods have (see Eakin and Brandenburger, 1970). Here, then, is a score for the conelike nature of the parietal receptors. Moreover, third eyes respond differently to different wavelengths of light (see Chapter 5). Cones are color receptors in lateral eyes.

This discussion has gone far enough, no doubt, to indicate that our knowledge is inadequate to classify the parietal-eye receptors of lizards. Although I once thought of them as conelike, the issue is presently less clear. It is better, in any event, to understand their structure and function than to be concerned over what we call them.

Moreover, it has been pointed out (Dodt, Ueck, and Oksche, 1971) that the type of photopigment and the nature of the neural connections in the retina are the bases of rod and cone reactions, not the structure of the outer segments. The presence of both rod and cone reactions is not at variance with the finding that only cells of one anatomical type are present.

Supportive Cells.

The receptor cells are surrounded by pigmented supportive cells; the two types, however, are not evenly distributed. Here and there each occurs in bundles. They are about equal in number, as determined by the ratio of their nuclei. I estimated a total of approximately 2,500 of each kind by dividing the area (15,000 μm^2) of the retina at the level of the inner segment by the cross-sectional area (3 μm^2) of a photoreceptor or a pigmented cell and dividing that number by two (Eakin, 1960). Both kinds of cells are cylindrical and have about the same diameter at the level selected for measurements.

Distally a supportive cell bears slender microvilli projecting into the lumen of the eye and alongside the bases of the receptoral processes. Occasionally one sees a stubby cilium embedded among the microvilli, evidence that the pigmented cells, like the receptors, are derived from ciliated cells (ependymal) lining the embryonic brain. Pigment granules, presumably of melanin, are abundant in the supportive cells, particularly in their distal halves. It has been noted previously that the pigment granules are shifted toward the lumen in light-adapted animals and basally in dark-adapted ones. The granules tend to be ovoid (2 by 0.5 μm) with their long axis in agreement with that of the cell. There are numerous microtubules, also longitudinally arranged, which may be involved in the pigment migration just mentioned. Supportive cells contain fewer mitochondria than do sensory cells.

At the level of the nuclei of the receptor cells the pigmented cells are narrow. If pigment granules are present in these stalklike regions, they are ordered in single file. Basally, the supportive cells broaden to become trumpets or foot-pieces that contact one another at points to form a meshed basket. The nucleus of a supportive cell usually resides in its foot-piece, which also contains considerable pigment.

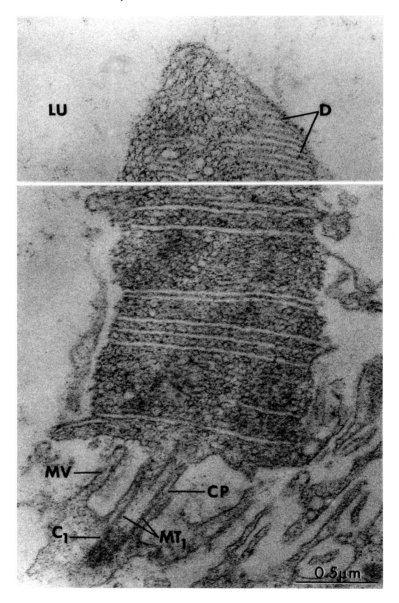

The distal ends of the supportive cells are joined by junctional complexes to receptor cells and to each other if two or more lie together in a bundle. Included in these complexes is a tight junction at the luminal surface, followed by an adhering zone, below which is a desmosome. The first-named is probably an important seal preventing the movement of molecules between the cells into or away from the lumen of the eye. The last-named organelle is thought to bind cells together, giving the retina internal strength. The desmosome is featured by very thick cell membranes, on the cytoplasmic sides of which are attached tufts of filaments. Additional binding of the cells together is achieved by fingerlike interdigitations along their lateral borders (Petit, 1968).

Ganglion Cells.

The third cell-type in the retina of the parietal eye is a large neurone called a ganglion cell, found below the level of the receptor cell nuclei but above the foot-pieces of the supportive cells. Ganglion cells are characterized by the following features: giant size, large nucleus, many mitochondria, and a perinuclear mass, termed Nissl substance, which is shown by electron microscopy to consist of strata or whorls of endoplasmic reticulum and by cytochemistry to be rich in ribonucleic acid (RNA).

The ganglion cells lie among the axons of the receptor cells with which they make synaptic contact, as described above. Axons lead from the ganglion cells, pass between the trumpets of the supportive cells, bundle with one another (Fig. 38), and enter the parietal nerve, to be described shortly. It is important to know the number of ganglion cells in an eye relative to the number of photoreceptors to determine the extent of summation or funneling—that is, the number of sensory cells connected functionally to a single ganglion cell. We have noted above that the number of photoreceptors in the third eye of *S. occidentalis* is approximately 2,500. How many ganglion

---

Fig. 37. EM of longitudinal section through third-eye receptor of *S. occidentalis* after long staining with osmium tetroxide. Tip and base of outer segment from two different receptors. c_1, distal centriole (kinetosome); CP, connecting piece; D, disks in outer segment; LU, lumen of eye; MT_1, ciliary microtubules (axoneme); MV, microvillus. $\times$ 44,000. Heretofore unpublished, Eakin, Brandenburger, and Ferlatte.

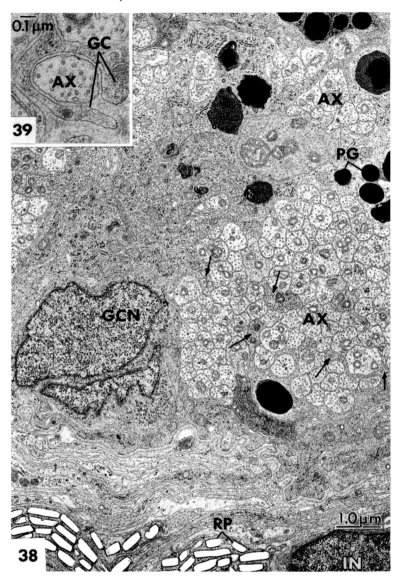

cells? I could not easily count them in sections of an eye, but the nerve fibers in the parietal nerve could be enumerated. The specimen shown in Figure 40 has 273 nerve fibers by actual count. Thus, approximately ten sensory cells synapse with each ganglion cell. The physiological significance of this conclusion will be discussed later.

The axons from the ganglion cells are assembled at the postero-ventral surface of the retina of the third eye in *S. occidentalis*. In other species the assembly point is midventral, as in *Sphenodon punctatus* or *Anguis fragilis*, described respectively by Dendy (1911) and by Nowikoff (1910) and Petit (1968). The fibers bundle (fasciculate), become embedded in glial cells (Fig. 38), and pass through the capsule of the eye to emerge as the parietal nerve. The glial cells, which enclose the ganglionic axons as they leave the retina, are probably modified supportive cells derived from the embryonic optic vesicle. They might be sheath cells, however, derived from neural crest cells which rode the tops of the neural folds when the primordium of the brain was formed. A third, but less likely, alternative is a mesodermal origin. Each glial or sheath cell supports many ganglionic axons by wrapping itself around the fibers and pulling them into the interior of the cell, maintaining, however, the integrity of its plasma membrane (Fig. 39). The axons thus only appear to be embedded within a supporting cell, the cytoplasm (axoplasm) of the fiber being separated from the cytoplasm of the supporting cell by two membranes: that of the axon and that of glial or sheath cell.

PARIETAL NERVE.

The cable of ganglionic fibers leaves the eye and becomes the parietal nerve (Fig. 40). Sheath cells outside the eye form supportive ele-

---

Fig. 38. EM of retina of parietal eye of *S. occidentalis*, showing bundling of axons (AX) from ganglion cells and embedment of axons by glial cells. GCN, nucleus of glial cell; IN, nucleus of capsular iridocyte; PG, pigment granules in supportive cell; RP, reflecting platelets in iridocyte of capsule. Arrows indicate fingers of glial cell enclosing axons. × 12,000. Heretofore unpublished, Eakin, Brandenburger, and Ferlatte.

Fig. 39. Enlargement of axon (AX) being engulfed by glial cell (GC). Note folds of glial cell have almost surrounded axon, which contains many microtubules. × 44,000. Heretofore unpublished, Eakin and Brandenburger.

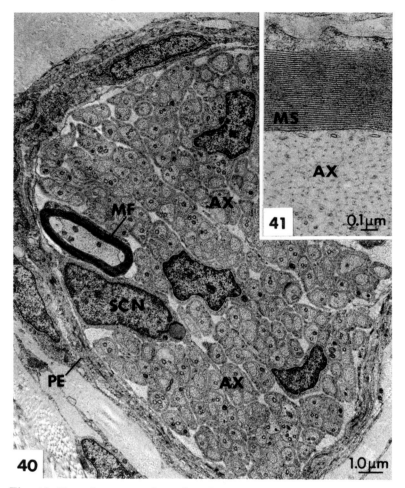

Fig. 40. Em of cross section of parietal nerve in *S. occidentalis*. AX, axons; MF, myelinated fiber; PE, capsule of nerve (perineurium); SCN, sheath cell nucleus. × 5,600. Heretofore unpublished, Eakin, Brandenburger, and Ferlatte.

Fig. 41. Enlargement of sector of myelin sheath (MS) of myelinated fiber in parietal nerve shown in Fig. 40. AX, cytoplasm (axoplasm) of axon. × 44,000. Heretofore unpublished, Eakin and Brandenburger.

ments along the course of the nerve. Any given cross section of the nerve usually reveals one or more sheath cells, recognized by their nuclei (SCN) and by some pigment granules in their cytoplasm (not illustrated). Neurites having a simple covering of sheath-cell membrane are said to be unmyelinated or nonmedullated. In *S. occidentalis* all fibers of the parietal nerve are of this kind (Eakin and Westfall, 1960), or so I thought until I recently made the picture shown here. I saw to my surprise one myelinated fiber (MF, Fig. 40), identified by the thick layer of concentric membranes which are visible only with an electron microscope (Fig. 41). This layer was called myelin by the light microscopist, who regarded it as a secretion of sheath cells or axons or both. The laminar investment is formed, we know now, by sheath cells making numerous revolutions about neurites. Oksche and Kirschstein (1968) found between 200 and 300 unmyelinated fibers in the parietal nerve of three European lizards, but in *Lacerta sicula* they observed myelinated fibers also (50 out of a total of 638), scattered among the nonmyelinated ones. A possible difference in function between the two types of fibers will be mentioned in Chapter 5.

The parietal nerve, after reaching the tip of the epiphysis, passes along the anterior surface of that organ, then swerves to the left side, continues to the base of the epiphysis, and enters the brain stem. Professor J. Ariëns Kappers of Amsterdam, a distinguished pinealogist, found precisely the same course of the parietal nerve in *Lacerta viridis* and showed that the nerve fibers enter a neural center (habenular ganglion) on the left (Kappers, 1965, 1967). This asymmetrical relationship of the parietal nerve has been reported in other reptiles: *Lacerta vivipara* by von Haffner (1953); *Anolis carolinensis* by Robert Ortman (1960), who was associated with Stebbins and me in the early days of our third-eye studies; and the tuatara, *Sphenodon punctatus*, by Dendy (1899, 1911). To me the most disturbing observation of right-handedness of the parietal nerve is that of Nowikoff (1910), for whose work I have great admiration. Von Haffner suggests that Nowikoff could have confused right and left sides of his sections. This is easily done. The ribbon of sections could have been mounted upside down, or the direction of sectioning of the specimens could have been the reverse of that assumed. But why this concern about right and left side? The sinistral relationship of the parietal nerve has important evolutionary significance, as we shall see in Chapter 4.

LENS.

The palisade of cells constituting the roof of the eye vesicle barely qualifies as a lens, which by definition is a light-refracting body by virtue of some quality, such as a curved surface. The so-called lens of the parietal eye of *S. occidentalis* is almost a flat plate (Fig. 26); the lower surface is slightly convex. In other species the lens is more globular. The cells are elongate cylinders, firmly knit together by interdigitating lateral surfaces, by desmosomes at their inner ends, and by the tightly adhering inner fibrous stratum of the cornea. The nuclei of the cells are basally situated but not all at the same level, giving the layer a pseudostratified feature.

The inner ends of the lens cells, bordering the lumen, bear microvilli, and from each cell a long cilium of $9 \times 2 + 2$ pattern (motile?) extends into the cavity of the eye. The cilia are a legacy from their embryonic origin, namely, the lining of the neural tube. Unlike the lenses of lateral eyes, which are skin lenses, those of the third eyes of reptiles are brain lenses! Electron microscopy and cytochemistry suggest that the inner zone of the lens cells, between nuclei and luminal border, is highly metabolic: denser cytoplasm; aggregations of mitochondria, glycogen granules, and secretory vesicles; and an accumulation of PAS-positive material and of RNA.

CAPSULE.

The eye is encased by a capsule on all sides, except above the lens, where its place is taken by the cornea. The capsule consists of a narrow, secreted layer (basal lamina) on the surface of the retina, a layer of connective tissue fibers (collagen) that appear banded in the electron microscope, and an external layer of highly specialized cells. We called those cells iridocytes (Eakin and Westfall, 1960) because they contain many rectangular crystals of light-refracting and reflecting material which impart a glistening appearance to the eye. The crystals often fracture and are lost when an eye is sectioned (see Fig. 42). At first, I assumed that the crystalline substance was guanine. My colleagues and I found, however, that these capsular cells were stainable with oil red O and oil blue N dyes, indicating the presence of lipids (Eakin, Quay, and Westfall, 1961). If an eye be fixed in formalin and then immersed in a lipid solvent, pyridine, at 60° C for twenty hours, the silvery appearance disappears and electron microscopy reveals a complete absence of the crystals, their places being marked by empty spaces. Curiously, in about one blue-bellied lizard in four the parietal eye lacks the silvery sheen. The coloration of the organ is dull black. The capsules of such eyes do not stain with oil red O, and they exhibit no crystals in the electron microscope. From these observations we concluded that the cells in question may contain both guanine and lipid. Petit (1968) does not describe the capsule in his EM study of the parietal eye of *Anguis fragilis*, but his Figure 1 shows the capsule to be a very thin encasement.

At the junction with the cornea, the capsule of the third eye is continuous with subcutaneous connective tissue (Fig. 26). It contains small blood vessels. The main blood supply to the reptilian parietal eye, based upon the studies of Dendy (1911) and Steyn (1958), is the anterior pineal artery, which is a branch of the posterior cerebral artery that in turn arises from the internal carotid artery. Blood flows forward in the anterior pineal artery and into the capillaries within the capsule of the eye and, according to Steyn, on the upper surface of the lens. Capillaries do not enter the retina, and the lens is also avascular. Venous blood from the eye is drained into the pineal vein, which encircles the eye, and empties into the longitudinal sinus (LS, Fig. 25), a large vascular sac enclosing the dorsal parts of the epiphysis and related organs. It is noteworthy that in *Sceloporus, Sphenodon* (Dendy, 1911), and several species of South African lizards (Steyn, 1958) the anterior pineal artery lies to the left of the midline of the body—another sinistral relationship.

CORNEA.

The skin above the eye is transparent, except during the molt of the scaly exoskeleton, when it is opaque. The transparency of this specialized region of the integument, the cornea, is owing to the

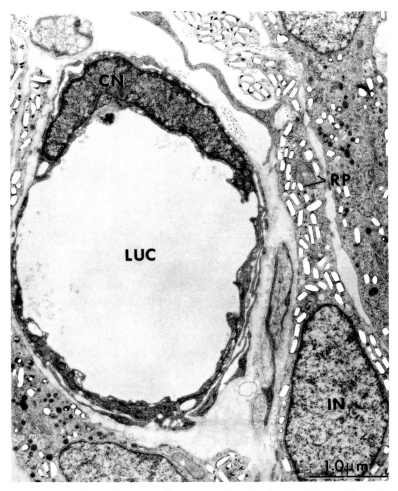

Fig. 42. EM of section through capsule of parietal eye of *S. occidentalis*. CN, nucleus of capillary cell; IN, nucleus of capsular cell (iridocyte); LUC, lumen of capillary; RP, reflecting platelets. × 9,000. Heretofore unpublished, Eakin and Brandenburger.

absence of melanophores (black pigmented cells), which are abundant elsewhere in the skin (Fig. 26), and to certain structural features such as close packing of the fibers of the innermost layer, absence of thick fibers in the middle spongy layer, and a tendency of cells and filaments within them to be oriented vertically. Above the cornea lies the thin, transparent interparietal scale, which is secreted by the cornea and surrounding skin. The scale is periodically shed (molt or ecdysis) and replaced by a new one.

In the living blue-belly the cornea has a yellowish color. It is not known whether the color is due to chromatophores or free pigment or to some structural feature of the cornea that reflects the yellow region of the visible spectrum. It may function as an interference filter.

MISCELLANEOUS.

In the lumen of the reptilian third eye may be seen large cells with pseudopodia, vesicles of digestive enzymes (lysosomes), residual bodies (remnants of intercellular digestion), and many inclusions, such as pigment granules and cellular debris. I identified these cells as macrophages, the scavengers of the body. On this point Petit (1967, 1968) concurs and adds the important observation that they contain stacks of membranes which, as noted above, are engulfed fragments of the outer segments of photoreceptors.

One frequently sees giant round or oval cells filled with pigment granules within the retina, usually peripherally. They were first noted by Steyn (1959*b*, 1960) in *Cordylus polyzonus*; we found them in *S. occidentalis* (Eakin, Quay, and Westfall, 1961); and Petit (1968) has recently observed them in *Anguis fragilis*. Their significance is not known.

Amphibian Third Eye

Having presented a moderately detailed account of the fine structure of the third eye of my leading character, I shall make the descriptions of the median eyes of frog and lamprey relatively brief. The title of this section is a misnomer for two reasons. First, not all amphibians have the third eye. Salamanders lack it. Moreover, it is missing in the adults of some frogs, including the Pacific Treefrog *Hyla regilla*, although they possess it as tadpoles. In the second place, even the best amphibian frontal organ can scarcely be termed an eye. It is a big step down in organization from the parietal eye of lizards.

A LITTLE HISTORY.

The parietal organ of frogs has been known for more than a century. It was discovered in 1865 by Ludwig Stieda, then an instructor (*Privatdozent*) at the University of Dorpat, Estonia. He noted a clearing in the skin of a frog (*Rana temporaria*) in the midline of the head at the level of the anterior border of the lateral eyes. He called it a brow spot (*Stirnfleck*). It not only lacked pigment cells but also integumentary glands. Under the brow spot Stieda found a spherical body about 0.15 mm in diameter, which he termed a frontal gland (*Stirndrüse*), believing that it must be some kind of secretory structure. De Graaf reported, in a work (1886) cited earlier, that Stieda's organ occurred in several European frogs and toads but not in a treefrog, *Hyla arborea*. It was Franz Leydig (1890), the discoverer of the reptilian parietal eye, who provided the first good description of Stieda's organ with informative drawings of it, showing internal cavity, blood supply, and innervation. Leydig remarked that although it had been called a gland by earlier workers he believed that the body could be placed in the category of an integumentary sense organ.

By 1905, when Studnička's aforementioned classic book appeared, several studies on the frontal organ had been conducted. To a valuable review of these works Studnička added his own observations, including that of rodlike projections from the inner ends of cells which he regarded as sensory in function. From 1905 until the advent of the electron microscope in biology, anatomical treatises on the amphibian stirnorgan (a term which we have adopted from the German, although we do not capitalize it) were more widely spaced in time than previously. The Swedish zoologist Nils Holmgren (1918) made a careful study of the living organ colored with dyes which do not kill the cells (vital staining) and of sections of specimens preserved by a variety of methods. He described three kinds of cells: sensory, epithelial or supportive, and ganglion. The receptoral process of the first-named was analyzed into outer and inner segments and likened to rods and cones of the lateral eye. Holmgren even figured cross or spiral banding of the outer segment—an approximation to the disks which only electron microscopy can clearly reveal (resolve). He found considerable variation in the appearance of the outer segments, which he attributed to cyclical phases of regeneration and degeneration, a conclusion which Riech (1925) and Winterhalter (1931) were unable to confirm. Kleine (1929) disagreed also with Holmgren's description of the sensory cell, including the analogy to outer and inner segments of lateral-eye receptors.

Twenty years after the publication of the papers by Kleine and Winterhalter another noteworthy work on the structure of the amphibian stirnorgan appeared. Andreas Oksche (1952), now professor of anatomy at the Justus Liebig University in Giessen, Germany, and a leading scholar on pineal organs, utilized new cytological procedures in his study of the frontal organ of a frog, *Rana temporaria*—the same form used by most of the earlier workers. Oksche restored confidence in Holmgren's analysis of the receptoral process, although at that time he doubted its sensory function, and he suggested the possibility of a relationship of the frontal organ to the pigmentation of the animals, a concept I shall explore in Chapter 5.

Next came the several studies using electron microscopy (Eakin, 1961; Eakin and Westfall, 1961; Oksche and von Harnack, 1962, 1963; Eakin, Quay, and Westfall, 1963; Kelly and Smith, 1964; and Kelly, 1965, 1971) upon which the following account is largely based.

GENERAL MORPHOLOGY.

A light micrograph (Fig. 43) of the third eye from a larva of *Hyla regilla* reveals the features mentioned in the introduction: an irregular lumen (LU), of which only the main chamber and left-hand arm appear in the section photographed; a thin roof composed of a single layer of cells; and a thick floor, the retina. As in the retina of the parietal eye of lizards, there are three cell types in the stirnorgan of amphibians: sensory, supportive, and ganglion. Cell boundaries are not discernible in Figure 43. The nuclei bordering the median and lateral arms of the lumen (see Fig. 4) belong to sensory and supportive cells. The large nuclei labeled GN are probably those of ganglion cells. The light non-nucleated areas (NF) are tangles

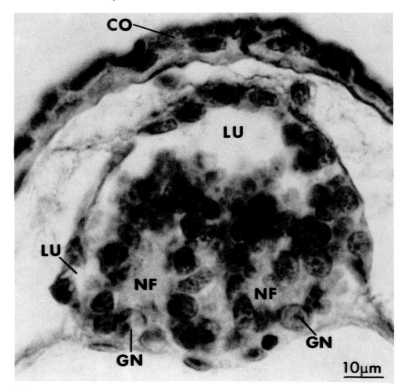

Fig. 43. LM of cross section of frontal organ in tadpole of *Hyla regilla*. CO, cornea; GN, nuclei of ganglion cells; LU, lumen of organ; NF, areas of nerve fibers (neuropile). × 1,000. From Eakin, Quay, and Westfall (1963).

(neuropile) of axons from receptor cells and dendrites from ganglion cells. The nerve fibers cannot be individually seen in this micrograph. The entire organ is encapsulated with a thin layer of flattened cells. Those on the ventral surface of the organ are a part of the covering (meninges) of the brain, those above are continuous with the dermis of the skin.

ELECTRON MICROSCOPY.

In an electron micrograph of the photoreceptor from the third eye of *H. regilla* (Fig. 44) one observes that the outer segment of a process is a stack of disks, 50 to 150 in number, which are patent to the lumen of the organ, as are the disks in the third eyes of lizards (Fig. 28). The $9 \times 2 + 0$ assembly of microtubules (MT_1) is likewise the same. A cross section through the connecting piece (Fig. 45) clearly shows the absence of central singlets and the enzyme-containing arms that occur on the doublets of motile cilia (Fig. 8). On the other hand, there is a greater variation in the form of the outer segment in the stirnorgan of amphibians than in that of the parietal eye of lizards. Well-ordered receptors, like the one shown in Figure 44, are the exception. Many outer segments are bent, contorted, and fragmented. Sometimes an outer segment is a whorl of membranes unconnected to the ciliary shaft from which they undoubtedly arose. The significance of this variability in relation to Holmgren's suggestion of a secretory activity of the frontal organ will be discussed later.

The inner segment of the process is similar to that of parietal-eye receptors of *Sceloporus* except for two particulars: (1) the absence or near-absence of a striated rootlet leading from the centrioles (c_1 and c_2) and (2) a greater number of mitochondria. Figure 44 illustrates a typical concentration of mitochondria in an inner segment, which in this instance extends up along one side of the outer segment. The dark dots in the mitochondria are called mitochondrial granules. They are found in many types of tissue, and they vary in composition from deposits of calcium, strontium, and barium to accumulations of iron, silver, and even gold! The small granules in the cytoplasm are ribosomes, the large ones glycogen.

The body of a sensory cell contains a relatively large nucleus, a prominent stack of cisternae (Golgi apparatus) in which secretions are packaged into vesicles, supranuclear aggregations of mitochondria, glycogen granules, and massive bundles of fine filaments which arise in the inner segment, curve around the nucleus, and enter the axon of the cell.

The axons of the sensory cells are usually short, broad processes which extend into tangles of nerve fibers (neuropile) near the ventral surface of the retina. The terminals of the axons (T, Fig. 46) contain mitochondria, the aforementioned filaments, masses of granules, and aggregations of synaptic vesicles. Synapses between these axonal enlargements and the dendrites of ganglion cells can be identified,

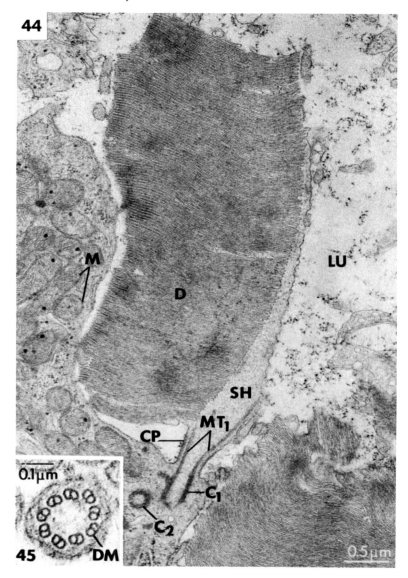

as in the parietal eye of *Sceloporus*, by local concentrations of synaptic vesicles adjacent to a thickened axonal membrane and by dark lines or bars, the synaptic ribbons (SNR, Fig. 47) oriented perpendicularly to the membrane. Sometimes two, or even three, synaptic ribbons occur adjacent to one another; the ribbons may be quite long (0.33 µm). At these synapses neural impulses pass from sensory cells to ganglion cells. Additionally, I have observed large, opaque bodies (OB, Fig. 46) with dense crystalline cores in the receptor terminals. The significance of these structures is unknown. Why, then, do I mention them? Just to indicate that there are still more worlds to explore and conquer. Kelly and Smith (1964) observed another type of apparent synapse in the frontal organ of the frog *Rana pipens*, namely, one in which the synaptic ribbon is lacking but where instead there is a flat synaptic cistern parallel to the axonal membrane.

Supportive cells (also called epithelial cells by Holmgren, 1918, and ependymal cells by Oksche and von Harnack, 1963) are scattered among the sensory cells. They appear to be homologous with the pigmented cells in the retina of the reptilian third eye. Pigment granules are present, at least in some forms, although they are few in number; slender microvilli and cilia (one per cell) project from the distal ends of the cells into the lumen of the organ; and basally the cells have foot-pieces like trumpets. Stout desmosomes bind the supportive cells to one another and to the sensory cells, and bundles of filaments probably give internal support. The presence of stacks of smooth cisternae, much rough endoplasmic reticulum, and many vesicles and vacuoles suggest synthetic activities. Finally, these cells possess internal, fusiform bodies composed of membranes (Eakin, Quay, and Westfall, 1963; Kelly and Smith, 1964), which are specializations of the endoplasmic reticulum. One is reminded of

---

Fig. 44. EM of longitudinal section of photoreceptoral process from frontal organ of *H. regilla*. c_1, distal centriole (kinetosome); c_2, proximal or accessory centriole; CP, connecting piece; D, disks of outer segment; LU, lumen of organ; M, mitochondria in inner segment; MT_1, microtubules of cilium (outer segment); SH, shaft of cilium. × 23,000. Heretofore unpublished, Eakin and Brandenburger.

Fig. 45. EM of cross section of connecting piece of photoreceptor in frontal organ of *H. regilla*. DM, doublet of microtubules. × 86,000. Heretofore unpublished Eakin and Brandenburger.

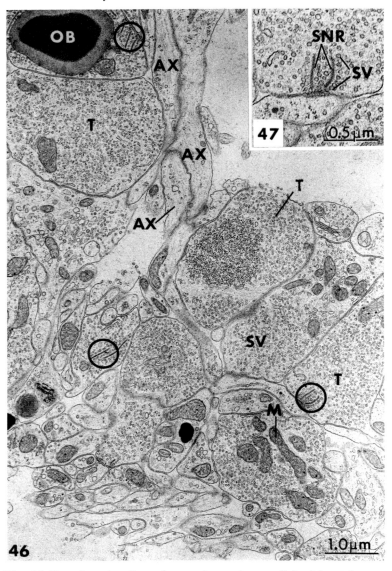

Fig. 46. Em of section through neural area (neuropile) of frontal organ of *H. regilla*. AX, axons of sensory cells; M, mitochondrion; OB, opaque body; SV, synaptic vesicles; T, axon terminals. Several synapses are encircled. × 14,000. From Eakin, Quay, and Westfall (1963).

Fig. 47. Enlargement of one of the synapses encircled in Fig. 46. SNR, synaptic ribbons; SV, synaptic vesicles. × 18,000.

similar bodies (myeloid) in the pigmented epithelium of certain vertebrate lateral eyes and of the possibility that these structures are light-sensitive.

Ganglion cells are large elements, like those in a reptilian parietal eye, situated in or adjacent to the masses of nerve fibers just described. Light microscopists identified them by their giant nuclei (4 to 7 μm) with a prominent internal density (nucleolus), by their small number (2 to 30 per organ), and by their staining reactions (see Oksche, 1952). Like most ganglion cells elsewhere, these cells possesses characteristic cytoplasmic granular regions (Nissl bodies) which stain with basic dyes. Electron microscopy reveals them to be concentrations of rough endoplasmic reticulum and ribosomes. Pigment granules may also be present. Dendrites of the ganglion cells synapse with the terminals of the receptor cells, as noted above, and an axon leads from the base of each ganglion cell into the frontal nerve.

The frontal nerve or frontal tract emerges from the posteroventral surface of the stirnorgan after passing through its thin capsule, continues through the subcutaneous connective tissue, enters the cranium between the parietal and frontal bones, and penetrates the epiphysis. The composition of the nerve in frogs has been studied by several German workers. The significant findings are as follows: the nerve contains a variable number of both myelinated and non-myelinated fibers (for example, 1 to 22 of the former, 35 to 146 of the latter, according to Oksche and Vaupel-von Harnack, 1965); the number of myelinated fibers agrees well with that of large ganglion cells in the frontal organ; the number of fibers of both kinds decreases as the nerve courses toward the epiphysis (reason unknown); the number of fibers which originate in the frontal organ and continue in the pineal tract leading from epiphysis to the brain is greatly reduced (to perhaps only 2 to 4 percent of the total), indicating that many fibers terminate in the epiphysis; and, last, there are some fibers (efferent) which carry nervous impulses to the eye (see Ueck, Vaupel-von Harnack, and Morita, 1971).

Why, the reader may ask, do I begin the above paragraph with frontal nerve or tract? Incidentally, some call the structure the pineal nerve. To the nonprofessional, biology seems unnecessarily cluttered with terminology. Indeed, some biologists—especially anatomists—

appear at times to be obsessed with semantics. We are only trying to make our science as precise as we can, being unable, usually, to describe the living world with numbers, formulae, and equations. Although we frequently speak of frontal. or parietal *nerves* from third eyes and optic *nerves* from lateral eyes, we should use the term *tracts*. A nerve is a cable of fibers outside the central nervous system (CNS, the brain and spinal cord in vertebrates), whereas a tract is a bundle of fibers within the CNS. You may reply, however, that median and lateral eyes lie outside the brain. But the retinas of these eyes are actually parts of the brain which become separated from the central nervous system in development, as I shall detail in the next chapter. Accordingly, the bundle of axons from the ganglion cells of the stirnorgan constitute a tract, passing from one part of the brain to another. Trivia? That may depend upon whether one is a student or a professor.

Third Eyes of Fishes

My third character, the lamprey, now claims the spotlight. If the taxonomist will kindly turn his head the other way—which may be asking too much—I shall lump the lampreys (cyclostomes) with the fishes in this chapter. We noted in the introduction that the lamprey's not one but two median eyes, the pineal and parietal, lie forward in the head (Fig. 5) in roughly the same position as that of the frontal organ of amphibians. Both are hollow bodies without lenses (Fig. 6); the parietal vesicle lies beneath and slightly to the left of the pineal one.

IN RETROSPECT.

Early zoologists, led by curiosity about the living world, took note of a silvery body on the top of the brain of lampreys, which was clearly visible through a transparent area of skin (Fig. 5). Included among these scientists was the distinguished Johannes Müller. Some examined the body microscopically and found that it was double but drew the erroneous conclusion that the two vesicles were only sub-divisions of one organ. It was not until 1893 that Studnička, a familiar name by now, demonstrated that each vesicle was independent of the other anatomically and developmentally. To the upper one he assigned the name *pineal organ* because it was an extension of the pineal body, or epiphysis. The lower one he called the parapineal organ (from the Greek *para*, meaning 'along side of'), which term is still in good standing. I am using *parietal*, however, for the sake of simplicity and to emphasize the similarity in the developmental origin (homology) of this vesicle and that of the parietal eye of lizards. Other studies quickly followed Studnička's, notably a work in 1894 by Carl von Küpffer, an anatomist at Munich. Von Küpffer is better known for the discovery of large, starlike cells in the liver, Kupffer cells, which remove debris and foreign bodies from the bloodstream. Between 1905 and the 1960s only two works on lamprey third eyes merit citation: a study by Dendy (1907), whom we met in connection with the median eye of the tuatara, and one by the Russian D. Tretjakoff (1915) of Odessa. The latter author described and figured the outer part of the sensory process as a kind of "hat which is composed of extraordinarily fine lamellae." Think of this quotation when you come to the picture revealed by electron microscopy (Fig. 50)!

The distinguished zoologist and anatomist Professor J. Z. Young of University College, London, demonstrated (1935) that light directed upon the pineal apparatus of a lamprey stimulated movements of the animal, although ablation of the organs did not abolish the response. Finally, the application of electron microscopy in biology led to new discoveries on the pineal and parietal vesicles of lampreys. Dr. Jane Westfall and I were apparently the first to see the ciliary photoreceptors in these organs (Eakin, 1963). We studied ammocoetes larvae of *Petromyzon marinus*, which we obtained from a supplier in Pennsylvania. We never completed our study, however, because of the temptation to explore the ultrastructure of invertebrate photoreceptors. Meanwhile, Jean-Pierre Collin and Annie Meiniel of Clermont-Ferrand, France, have produced several splendid papers on the pineal and parietal organs of another lamprey, *Lampetra planeri* (see Collin, 1969*b*, and Meiniel, 1971, for references to their works). The following account is based largely upon the investigations of Collin and Meiniel plus our unpublished observations, including a recent look at the pineal organs of a West

Coast lamprey, *Entosphenus tridentatus*, by Jean Brandenburger, Millie Miller Ferlatte, and me.

GENERAL MORPHOLOGY.

The light micrograph shown in Figure 48 is of a longitudinal section through the two eye vesicles (PI, pineal; PA, parietal) of the ammocoetes of *E. tridentatus* (Fig. 6). Dorsal lies to the reader's right instead of at the top as in previous figures. The integument, the thin fibrous cranial roof, and the connections of the organs to epiphysis and brain were removed at the time of fixation. The pineal eye is a slightly flattened, ovoid, hollow body with a relatively thin roof and a thick floor. The former is composed of cuboidal or cylindrical cells. Aggregations of them project into the lumen of the vesicle, making the under surface of the roof very irregular. Studnička (1905) stated that the dorsal wall of the vesicle, which he called a pellucida (clear layer), reminded him of a lens, although he added that he did not suggest that it so functioned. It seems to me highly unlikely that it serves as a lens, at least in the ammocoetes of *E. tridentatus*.

The retina contains the same three types of cells encountered in amphibian and reptilian median eyes: sensory, supportive, and ganglion. Prominent processes project into the cavity of the vesicle from the distal ends of the sensory cells. With the knowledge of their fine structure from electron microscopy one can identify with confidence both inner segments (IS) and outer segments (OS) of these receptoral processes (Fig. 48). The former are bulbous or cylindrical projections from the retinal surface; the latter appear as highly irregular, often rounded bodies, seemingly lying free in the lumen of the organ. A diverticulum of the cavity often extends deep into the retina. A cross section of this canal is to be seen in Figure 48 (see arrow). Studnička referred to it as an atrium. Receptoral processes extend into the lumen of this recess. The supportive cells are distinguished by a large number of small granules in their cytoplasm. Ganglion cells (G) with lightly staining cytoplasm and large nuclei are situated at or near the base of the retina. The spaces between cells are probably artifacts of preservation.

The parietal vesicle is smaller and more rotund than the pineal

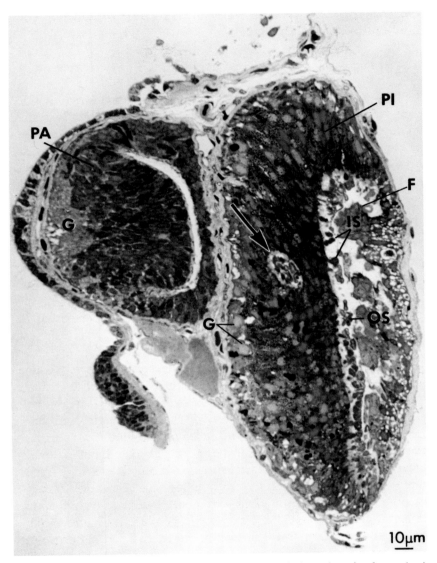

Fig. 48. Lᴍ of longitudinal section of pineal eye (ᴘɪ) and parietal eye (ᴘᴀ) from young ammocoetes of *E. tridentatus*. Dorsal aspect to reader's right. ғ, fold in roof of pineal eye; ɢ, ganglion below parietal eye, also two ganglion cells in pineal eye; ɪs, inner segments of pineal receptoral processes; os, outer segments of pineal receptoral processes. Arrow indicates recess (atrium) of lumen of pineal eye. × 480. Heretofore unpublished, Eakin and Blaker.

vesicle. Its lumen is strongly convex; its roof is thin at the center but thick on the sides. The upper wall is called by Meiniel (1971) an inverted retina because it possesses sensory processes which project backward away from the incoming light. I speculate that the distal wall of the parietal vesicle would be a clear, nonretinal layer like the tops of other median eyes if the organ had not become covered by the pineal vesicle in the course of evolution. The thick, arched floor of the parietal vesicle is a converse or uninverted retina because its sensory processes project forward into the cavity, as in the parietal eyes of lizards and in the frontal organs of amphibians. The retina is composed of at least three types of cells: sensory, supportive, and ganglion. Beneath the retina lies a body, a ganglion (G), which is either a part of or intimately related to a center (left habenular ganglion) in the brain (see Studnička, 1905, and Meiniel and Collin, 1971). A ganglion differs from a tangle of nerve fibers (neuropile). The former possesses nuclei of nerve cells; the latter has only axons and dendrites. Synapses occur in both, as do glial cells, the connective tissue cells of the nervous system.

ELECTRON MICROSCOPY OF LAMPREY PINEAL EYE.

In view of the general similarity of the lamprey's third eyes to those of *H. regilla* and *S. occidentalis*, I shall limit this description to features unique to cyclostomes. An electron micrograph (Fig. 49) of a small region of the pineal vesicle of *E. tridentatus* shows the large amount of "stuff" in the cavity of the-organ (LU). The whorls and stacks of membranes (OS) are cast-off outer segments of receptoral processes which one can see in the light microscope (Fig. 48). Inner segments (IS) of the sensory processes extend remarkably far into the cavity of the organ. They are packed with mitochondria and ribosomes. Additionally, the lumen contains short microvilli from both sensory and supportive cells (SC) and debris. A "regular" outer segment with its disks attached to a ciliary shaft is shown in Figure 50. The disks are unusually large in diameter (10 to 15 μm). In other dimensions, spacing, and patency with the lumen they resemble the disks of cones of lateral eyes. The outer segments are usually arched or wavy, probably because of the large size of the disks. The number of disks is lower than that in other median eyes,

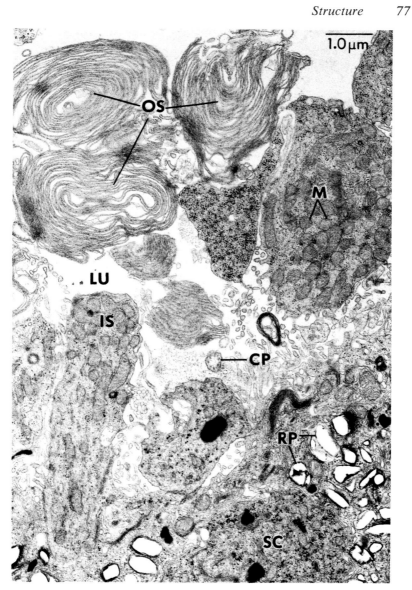

Fig. 49. EM of section through part of pineal vesicle of *E. tridentatus*. CP, connecting piece of receptor; IS, inner segment; LU, lumen of vesicle; M, mitochondria; OS, outer segments; RP, reflecting platelets (fractured); SC, supportive cell. × 12,000. Heretofore unpublished, Eakin and Brandenburger.

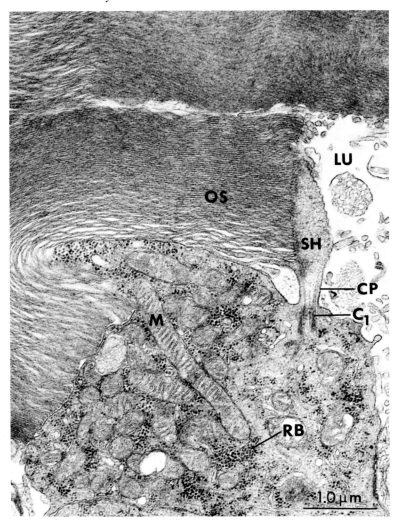

Fig. 50. Em of longitudinal section through photoreceptor in pineal eye of *E. tridentatus*. C_1, distal centriole (kinetosome); CP, connecting piece; LU, lumen of vesicle; M, mitochondrion; OS, outer segment (another outer segment lies above); RB, ribosomes; SH, shaft of outer segment (cilium). × 20,000. Heretofore unpublished, Eakin and Brandenburger.

although I have counted as many as 175 in ammocoetes of *Petro-myzon marinus*. According to Collin (1969*a*), the number of disks in the pineal eye of *Lampetra planeri* ranges from 30 to 130. Figure 51 illustrates another outer segment—call it irregular—which seems to be in the process of sloughing its disks. Still other outer segments appear to consist of only the dilated base of a ciliary shaft with or without a few short disks. Collin (1969*a, b*) stated that these receptors had aspects of rudimentary structures. I think that there is a good possibility that such processes have just lost their disks and are at the beginning of a regenerative phase (see Chapter 5).

A cross section of the connecting piece (CP, Fig. 52) of a sensory process reveals the familiar ring of nine doublets of microtubules. Fine bridges, or spokes, appear to connect the doublets to the membrane of the connecting piece. In some doublets the material within one microtubule appears dark, whereas the other tubule is clear. The same feature is to be seen in the doublets of a blue-belly's third-eye receptor (Fig. 10). I do not know the significance of this feature. The membrane of the connecting piece is fluted, indicating nine longitudinal ridges on the surface of this part of the process. Most of the above details were first noted by Collin (1969*a*).

There is nothing about the rest of the sensory cell upon which I wish to comment. Its structure is diagramed in Figure 53, which I have taken, with simplification, from Collin's monograph (1969*b*). It is noteworthy that the synapses between axons of receptor cells and dendrites of ganglion cells have the same features as those in other median eyes, namely, synaptic ribbons surrounded by synaptic vesicles. Sometimes there are as many as six synaptic ribbons in a row. The supportive cells (SC, Fig. 49) are unique in one important aspect: they contain reflecting platelets, which are responsible for the silvery appearance of the organ (see Fig. 5). In the light microscope these appear as dots stained darkly with methylene blue (Fig. 48), but in the electron microscope they are seen as empty vacuoles (RP, Fig. 49). In cutting ultrathin sections, the substance or substances of the platelets became fractured and dislodged, frequently leaving only the bounding membranes. The platelets are variable in size, shape, and position, unlike the uniform rectangular and semi-oriented platelets in the capsule of the parietal eye of *Sceloporus* (Fig. 42). Meiniel (1971) has made an excellent study of these

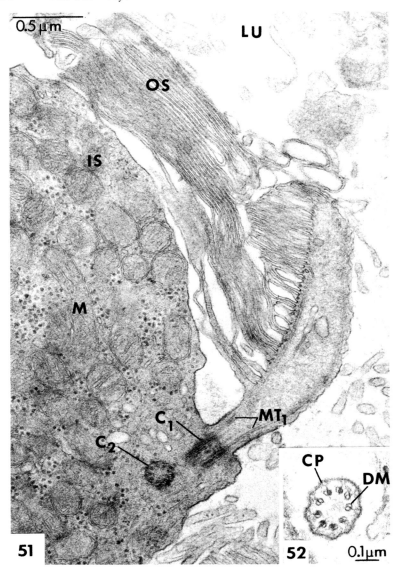

51

52

bodies—she calls them crystalline vacuoles—in the pineal and parietal eyes of *Lampetra planeri*. Incidentally, she finds them only in the dorsal retina of the parietal vesicle and there in relatively small numbers in comparison with the high concentration of them in the retina of the pineal vesicle. On the basis of several tissue-chemical tests (histochemistry) and the appearance of the vacuoles in light vibrating in one plane (polarized light) she concludes that the crystalline material in the vacuoles is guanine, a compound commonly found in reflecting layers of eyes, both vertebrate and invertebrate. This same compound, by the way, is one of the building blocks of our hereditary material (DNA), but our genes do not sparkle.

Ganglion cells lie near the lower surface of the retina of the pineal vesicle (Figs. 48, 53). They have large nuclei, masses of endoplasmic reticulum and ribosomes, synaptic contacts with receptor cells, and axons which leave the eye and pass to the epiphysis as the pineal tract.

ELECTRON MICROSCOPY OF LAMPREY PARIETAL EYE.

The fine structure of the parietal vesicle is like that of the pineal eye in most particulars. We have already noted that Meiniel (1971) found sensory processes projecting into the lumen of the organ from its roof (dorsal retina) and that the reflecting platelets are much less abundant than in the pineal eye and occur in only the supportive cells of the roof. Incidentally, both of these points were made earlier by the Russian Tretjakoff (1915). The receptoral processes vary greatly in form, as do those of the pineal vesicle. Some are regarded by Meiniel as rudimentary.

Ganglion cells are sparse in number in the roof (on the anterior part only) and especially few in the ventral retina. Most of the

Fig. 51. EM of longitudinal section of photoreceptor in pineal vesicle of *E. tridentatus*, showing sloughing of disks. C_1, distal centriole (kinetosome); C_2, proximal or accessory centriole; IS, inner segment; LU, lumen of vesicle; M, mitochondrion; MT_1, microtubules (axoneme) of cilium; OS, outer segment. × 37,000. Heretofore unpublished, Eakin and Brandenburger.

Fig. 52. EM of cross section of connecting piece (CP) of receptor in pineal vesicle of *E. tridentatus*. DM, doublet of microtubules. × 56,000. Heretofore unpublished, Eakin, Brandenburger, and Ferlatte.

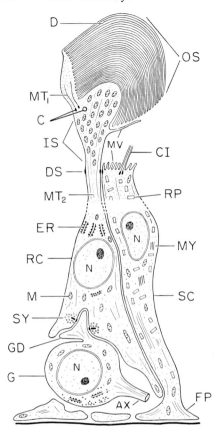

Fig. 53. Diagram of sensory (RC), supportive (SC), and ganglion (G) cells in pineal eye of lampreys. Sections deleted from cells indicated by dashed lines. AX, axon of ganglion cell; C, centrioles (distal and proximal); CI, unmodified cilium (kinocilium) of supportive cell; D, disks; DS, desmosome (cell contact); ER, rough endoplasmic reticulum (with ribosomes); FP, foot-piece of supportive cell; GD, dendrite of ganglion cell; IS, inner segment of receptoral process; M, mitochondrion; MT$_1$, microtubules (axoneme) of cilium; MT$_2$, cytoplasmic microtubules; MV, microvilli; MY, stack of cytoplasmic membranes (myeloid body); N, nuclei; OS, outer segment; RP, reflecting platelet; SY, synapse with synaptic ribbon and synaptic vesicles. Simplified from Collin (1969*b*); Emily E. Reid, delineator.

ganglion cells of the latter lie in the parapineal ganglion beneath the parietal vesicle (Meiniel, 1969; Meiniel and Collin, 1971).

In addition to the usual types of cells in median eyes, Collin (1969*a, b*) and Meiniel (1971) believe that there is another kind in both pineal and parietal vesicles, which they call cells with residual bodies. The chief identifying feature is the presence of dense bodies composed of whorls of membranes. They suggest the possibility that these cells engulf (phagocytose) cast-off parts of other cells. I am inclined to view these cells as variations of the supportive type, although I have not studied lamprey eyes sufficiently to make a judgment.

PINEAL AND PARIETAL ORGANS OF FISHES.

The true fishes will be slighted in my story because they, among lower vertebrates, have the least eyelike pineal organ, albeit in many the expanded tip of the epiphysis lies just beneath the skin and a thin region in the cranial roof, and the cells which line its lumen are clearly photoreceptors, anatomically and physiologically. The early studies on fish pineals, which began in the late 1880s, are summarized in Studnička's (1905) splendid monograph and again by Tilney and Warren (1919). Studnička added his own observations on pineal organs in representatives of sharks, rays, and chimeras (Chondrichthyes), a group of archaic fishes (Palopterygi), and modern bony fishes (Neoptergyi). For references to later works, including electron microscopy, the reader is referred to papers by the German investigators Oksche and Kirschstein (1967) and the Swedish zoologists Claes Rüdeberg (1969*b*) and Owman and Rüdeberg (1970).

In most instances the epiphysis in fishes is a long tube from the roof of the brain. In a dogfish, *Scyliorhinus canicula*, which Rüdeberg (1969*b*) studied, the organ may be 16 mm in length. Only the last two millimeters constitute the end-vesicle, which is the counterpart of the pineal eye of lampreys. Although the integument and brain case are thin above the tip of the pineal organ, there is no pigment-free spot as in lampreys or amphibians. The sensory cells send forth receptoral processes into the lumen of the epiphysis; they are composed of typical outer and inner segments. The outer segment is a modified cilium with as many as 150 disks in the above-mentioned dogfish. Features already described in the more eyelike vesicles of other vertebrates characterize the end-vesicles of fish pineals: supportive and ganglion cells, areas of neural fibers (neuropile), synapses (with synaptic ribbons) between receptor terminals and dendrites of ganglion cells, and so forth. The axons from the ganglion cells traverse the long epiphysis to reach centers in the brain.

Finally, there is in some fishes a small parietal organ which is probably comparable (homologous) to the parietal eyes of other vertebrates. I surmise that a careful search would disclose a parietal organ in many fishes. In a rainbow trout, *Salmo gairdneri*, Claes Rüdeberg (1969*a*) finds the parietal (parapineal) organ to be a small mass of sensory, supportive, and ganglion cells situated to the left of the pineal organ and above the left habenular ganglion, to which it is connected by a bundle of nerve fibers (parapineal tract). The parietal organ contains a narrow cavity into which project disk-containing ciliary processes from the distal ends of the few sensory cells.

And so, somewhat anticlimatically, the curtain falls on the second act of my play. Act 3 will be another excursion into history—developmental history this time—or a chronology of events in the embryo leading to an adult third eye.

4

Development

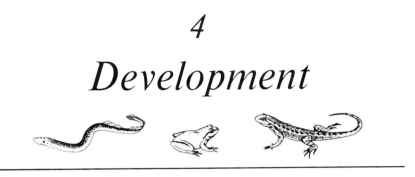

"Embryology can answer questions and solve perplexing anatomical riddles," I frequently say to my premedical students. It can help us find answers to such questions as why the receptors of a third eye project from the front surface of the retina, instead of extending from its back surface, as rods and cones in the lateral eyes do. What causes the skin above a third eye to become transparent? Why is the lens of the parietal eye derived from the brain and not the skin, as is the lens of a lateral eye? Does the parietal nerve originate in the brain or in the eye? Why is the eye associated with the left side of the brain? What is the evidence that the light-sensitive disks of outer segments are derived from a cilium? Indeed, what causes the cilium to form in the first place? And so forth.

Most anatomical studies cited in Chapter 3 included observations on embryonic as well as adult pineal and parietal eyes. Alexander Goette first noted that a third eye (of the Fire-bellied Toad *Bombinator igneus*) is derived from the brain (1873). It, like other third eyes, is formed from the dorsal wall of a region called the betwixt brain (diencephalon)—betwixt because it lies between cerebrum and cerebellum. The embryonic diencephalon of vertebrates develops several outpocketings: the two large lateral ones become the principal eyes, and one of the dorsal evaginations, the pineal diverticulum, is the source of the median eye (Fig. 54). To illustrate this story we return to our hero—correction, heroine—the female blue-bellied lizard, who, by the way, is not so blue as her mate.

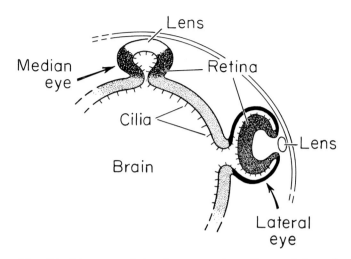

Fig. 54. Diagram of development of median and lateral eyes of vertebrates. From Eakin (1970); Emily E. Reid, delineator.

Formation of Median Optic Vesicle

A female *Sceloporus occidentalis* lays her eggs in a shallow depression which she digs in moist, well aerated soil. The breeding season, according to Stebbins (1954), is from May 15 to July 15. Since gravid females, collected in the late spring, will lay eggs in the laboratory, it is more economical of time to capture these animals than it is to search for their eggs in the field. Unfortunately, I do not possess the intuition of one of my good friends, Dr. Helen B. Jordan, who tells me that when she needs lizard's eggs for her malarial studies she simply asks herself, "If I were a female lizard, where would I lay my eggs?"

As mating occurs in the early spring, the female blue-bellies captured in May and June and brought to the laboratory oviposit fertile eggs; indeed, development is probably well begun at the time of laying. Upon opening the thin, flexible but tough eggshell, one finds the transparent embryo within some delicate membranes and attached to a large yolk sac filled with yellowish yolk, the embryo's store of nutrients. One can observe the pineal evagination by gently removing an early embryo of the right age, placing it in a dish of saline under a dissecting microscope, and illuminating it from the side. The pineal outpocketing looks like a small, clear bubble on the roof of the brain. Cross sections through the head of such an embryo yielded the photographs shown in Figures 55 through 58. The point of evagination of the pineal diverticulum from the brain may be seen in the first micrograph. The connection between the cavity (third ventricle) of the brain and the lumen of the outpocketing is indicated by the arrow.

The next micrograph (Fig. 56), of a section several micrometers farther anterior to that in the preceding figure, shows the posterior half of the diverticulum, which will later become the epiphysis. This organ will retain its embryonic position above the brain and the connection between its lumen and that of the diencephalon.

The section used for Figure 57 shows the anterior half of the diverticulum, the primordium of the parietal eye. Already future lens (L) can be distinguished from presumptive retina (R) by the elongate shape of the cells of the former. The cornea is represented at this stage by the outer embryonic layer (ectoderm) of flattened cells. Elements of the middle embryonic layer (mesoderm), which will form the deeper strata of the cornea, are just beginning to creep between the ectoderm and the prospective lens. The retina shows no clear structural differentiation, such as, for example, acquisition of pigment. At the biochemical level, however, certain cells are probably irreversibly determined to form sensory elements, others to be supportive in function, and still others to become ganglion cells. I call the reader's attention to the slightly asymmetrical shape of the lumen and to the position of "center of gravity" of the developing eye on one side of the midline of the brain (marked by the arrow). That side is *left*. The parietal eye has a slightly sinistral position in its early embryonic history.

Finally, Figure 58 is of a section taken through the constriction of the pineal diverticulum which, when complete, will subdivide the outpocketing into its two derivatives: the parietal eye from the anterior half and the epiphysis from the posterior half. The cavities of the two vesicles are still connected by a narrow canal. Careful examination of this photograph will reveal asymmetrical features: the canal lies to the left of the midline and so does the bulk of the parietal vesicle (PA), whereas the part of the epiphysis (EP) visible in this

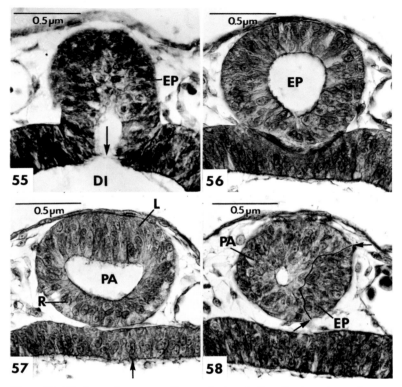

Figs. 55–58. LM of cross sections of pineal diverticulum in early embyro of *S. occidentalis*. Sequence of sections from posterior to anterior: Figs. 55, 56, 58, 57. DI, diencephalon of brain (note continuity of brain and pineal diverticulum, indicated by arrow in Fig. 55); EP, epiphysial part of diverticulum; L, incipient lens of parietal eye; PA, parietal part of diverticulum; R, retina. Arrow in Fig. 57 marks midline of embryo; arrows and line in Fig. 58 indicate boundary between epiphysial and parietal parts of diverticulum. × 700. Fig. 55. Heretofore unpublished, Eakin and Baker; Figs. 56–58, Eakin and Baker, from Eakin (1964*a*).

section is on the right side of the embryo (note arrows and line).

Now, why make a point of this asymmetry? Simply because it instructs us that the primordium of the parietal eye is "budded" from the left side of the pineal diverticulum. To state it differently, the plane of constriction which subdivides the diverticulum into anterior and posterior vesicles is not transverse but oblique, with the result that the former is shifted to the left, the latter to the right. This embryonic feature was not recognized until I chanced upon it (Eakin,

1964*a*), perhaps because most workers appear to have studied sagittal sections of early embryos of lizards, which do not reveal left-right relationships of parietal and pineal primordia so clearly as do transverse sections. Nowikoff (1910) illustrated cross sections of the pineal diverticulum of *Lacerta vivipara* (his Plate 3, Figs. 2 and 7), which look a little asymmetrical to me, but he made no comment on the feature. It should be added that there are instances of two transversely oriented pineal diverticula in early embryos of other vertebrates: fishes (Hill, 1891, 1894; Locy, 1894), amphibians (Cameron, 1903*a*), the tuatara (Dendy, 1911), and birds (Cameron, 1930*b*).

In Chapter 2, I presented very briefly the paleontological evidence of two pineal foramina in some ancient fishes, suggesting the presence of two third eyes in early vertebrates—pineal on the right, parietal on the left. Then in the description of third eyes of fishes I emphasized the slight sinistral position of the parietal vesicle in lampreys and its connection to a neural center (habenular ganglion) on the left side. I noted further that in some bony fishes (salmon and pike, for example) there is a parietal organ situated to the left of the epiphysis and connected to the left neural center. Additionally, I have already discussed the sinistral relationships of the parietal nerve in lizards and in the tuatara. Finally, there is an occasional secondary or accessory pineal body in birds (see Quay and Renzoni, 1967) which may represent a vestige of a left diverticulum. To summarize this digression: there are paleontological, anatomical, and embryological indications of an ancestral plan of paired median eyes.

Creation of Receptor

We know from the anatomy of the adult parietal eye receptor, presented in some detail in Chapters 1 and 3, that the light-sensitive apparatus is a modified cilium, but only the embryo can tell us how a cilium is formed and then transformed into an outer segment of the receptor. Until now this information on reptiles has not been available. Accordingly, Jean Brandenburger, Millie Miller Ferlatte, and I recently conducted new research for this chapter. The electron microscope enabled us to visualize the origin of the sensory apparatus in the embryonic pineal diverticulum of *S. occidentalis* and of the American Chameleon *Anolis carolinensis*.

Soon after the parietal vesicle has separated from the epiphysis by the constriction of the primary diverticulum, the centrioles within the cells lining the cavity migrate from the vicinity of the nuclei toward the luminal ends of the cells. Until this time the centrioles have been involved in cell divisions. Now, however, divisions cease in those cells which initiate differentiation into sensory, supportive, and lens types. In Figure 59 we observe the distal end of a young sensory cell and the first step in the formation of a receptoral process, the creation of the inner segment (is).

I believe that the inner segment is formed by a constriction below the tip of the sensory cell at the level of its attachments (j) to neighboring supportive cells. I speculate further that the constriction is produced by the contraction of fine fibrils embedded in the cytoplasm adjacent to the cell membranes at the junctions with supportive cells. Since the filaments are circularly oriented, we see them in cross-sectional view as fine dots. Their contraction, in the manner of a purse string, squeezes the distal end of the cell into the lumen to form the inner segment of the future receptoral process. This mechanism, if correct, would be similar to that postulated by my student Patricia C. Baker in her doctoral thesis (Baker, 1965) to explain the narrowing of embryonic cells when they invaginate (in gastrulation) to form the beginnings of a digestive tract. Later she and Thomas Schroeder (Baker and Schroeder, 1967) demonstrated the same mechanism for changing cell shape in the establishment of the embryonic nervous system (in neurulation). Perhaps the arrival of the centrioles in their upward migration from the nucleus is the stimulus for the contraction of the filaments.

The reader should note other features of developmental significance. A striated rootlet is beginning to form in association with the centrioles; microvilli project from the luminal surface of supportive and sensory cells; ribosomes (rb) are numerous in the cytoplasm of the inner segment (engaged in the synthesis of new proteins, one of which may be a photopigment?), and longitudinally arranged microtubules are abundant (involved in guiding raw materials into the inner segment?). The young process must be bubbling with metabolic activities preparatory to the formation of the ciliary outer segment.

In the sensory cell shown in the next photograph of the series (Fig. 60) the centrioles lie closer to the cell membrane, and the distal centriole appears to be "caught in the act" of stimulating the formation of a cilium. The plasma membrane has invaginated immediately above the centriole (black arrow), and between the centriole and membrane one can see strands of dark material (white arrow). The latter are incipient microtubules of the future cilium. There is a slight elevation of the membrane above these streamers. Had the embryo been fixed a few hours later, this elevation would have become a balloonlike evagination with an internal array of microtubules arranged in a ring of nine doublets—a young cilium. The second, or accessory, centriole (C_2) has taken its definitive position near and at right angles to the principal centriole (C_1). A part of a striated rootlet (SR) may be seen. Nearby sections show the connection of the rootlet to the centrioles. The rootlet will serve to anchor the cilium to the inner segment. The cytoplasmic microtubules (MT_2) may function as stiffeners or cell skeleton as well as channels for the movement of materials. The flow of substances is probably along the outer surfaces of the tubules instead of within their narrow lumens. The extracellular space between the halves of the cell junction (J, Fig. 60) is relatively clear and about 300 A wide. This kind of junction is technically called a *zonula adherens* (*zonula* because it is a band encircling the cell, and *adherens* because it serves to attach two adjacent cells to each other). The junction on the opposite side of the cell is a dark blur because the angle of section was tangential to the two cell membranes. Below a cell junction the intercellular space is clearer than that at the junction, and it looks like a meandering river because of the interdigitation of sensory and supportive cells. This interlocking further binds the cells together.

Would that I could set up a motion-picture camera inside the parietal eye vesicle to photograph the growing cilium. But I have only static electron micrographs—recordings of the state of development at moments in time. The gaps must be filled by imagination. The cilium rises and elongates; building materials—molecules of

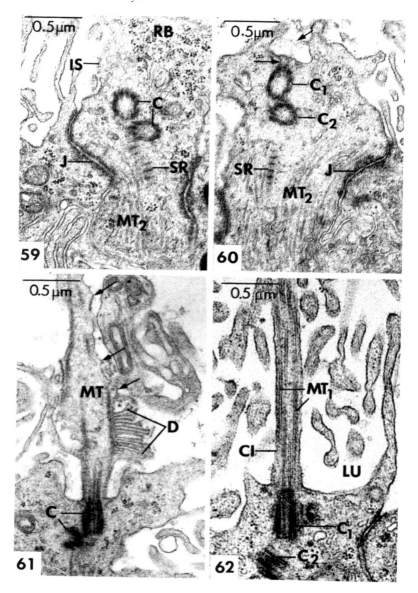

protein, lipid, and complex carbohydrates—stream out of the inner segment along the microtubules, which lengthen in pace with the growing ciliary membrane. Then a dramatic event occurs—the ciliary membrane folds sharply a few micrometers above the base of the cilium. Similar evaginations or pleats occur in rapid succession, so that the cilium is quickly transformed into an outer segment of a photoreceptor by the establishment of a stack of disks. Figure 61 illustrates a young outer segment in which the lowermost disks, the first to be formed, may be observed. At this time they are shorter, thicker, and more irregular than those of later stages (compare with the adult disks in Fig. 9). The distal part of the cilium has not yet formed disks, although there are slight indications (see arrows) of new diskal outgrowths.

Meanwhile, cilia are developing from the tips of supportive and lens cells, but they do not form disks (Fig. 62). They retain their cylindrical shape, and the pattern of their microtubules is $9 \times 2 + 2$. Why, the reader may ask, does one embryonic cell differentiate an elaborate sensory apparatus but no pigment, whereas its immediate neighbor forms an ordinary cilium and an abundance of pigment granules? Any embryologist would cry "Eureka!" if he discovered the answer. This is one of the major unsolved problems in developmental biology.

The process of disk formation continues in older processes by repeated outgrowths of the ciliary membrane at the base of the outer segment. One would not know this from inspection of electron micrographs of ciliary photoreceptors. Dr. Richard Young and his associates have conducted instructive experiments to demonstrate the basal origin of disks in retinal rods of lateral eyes (1970, 1971a). I assume that his findings apply also to median eyes of vertebrates. He ad-

---

Figs. 59–62. Stages in differentiation in the embryonic retina of the parietal eye of *S. occidentalis*. c, centrioles; c_1, distal centriole (kinetosome); c_2, proximal or accessory centriole; CI, unmodified cilium (kinocilium) of supportive cell; D, disks in very young outer segment; IS, inner segment; J, cell contact (zonula adherens); LU, lumen of eye; MT_1, microtubules (axoneme) of cilium; MT_2, cytoplasmic microtubules; RB, ribosomes; SR, striated rootlet. Upper arrow in Fig. 60 indicates invagination of cell membrane above kinetosome, lower arrow points to beginning of ciliary microtubules; arrows in Fig. 61 mark points of incipient evaginations of ciliary membrane to form disks. $\times$ 30,000. Heretofore unpublished, Eakin, Brandenburger, and Ferlatte.

ministered radioactive amino acids to salamanders, frogs, mice, rats, and monkeys, removed their eyes at varying times after injecting the tagged amino acid, and prepared them for autoradiography, as explained earlier. Young found that the administered amino acid is promptly taken up from the bloodstream by retinal rod cells; it moves up the inner segment; and then it appears in the lowermost disks, having been incorporated into proteins of the outer segment. Eyes of increasing age after injection showed a progressive shift of the radioactive disks to more and more distal levels in the outer segment. Why the shift? Because new unlabeled disks form at the base—one every forty minutes in frogs—and move the radioactive disks farther along the shaft of the outer segment.

Induction of Pineal Anlage

Before proceeding further with the story of development, I go back in time to discuss briefly an important event prior to the formation of the pineal diverticulum, namely, the induction of the pineal anlage. The general reader may find two new words in this subtitle. *Induction* is the term given to the influence of one part of an embryo (or transplant or even nonliving object) upon another part of the embryo, resulting in the development of the latter into a particular type of cell or tissue. Induction is a twentieth-century contribution to principles of developmental biology stemming from the analysis of extensive experimentation, such as removal, transplantation, and culture of embryonic cells. The development of the embryonic district which has been influenced by the inductor is said to be dependent. For example, ectoderm is dependent upon influences, chiefly chemical substances, from underlying mesoderm for differentiation into nervous tissue, sense organs, and certain glands.

The word *anlage* (plural, *anlagen*), as used in developmental biology, refers to an early embryonic district which will form a specific structure. We speak of the anlage of a limb or thyroid gland or pineal diverticulum. The word is German, with several meanings, including a tax! There is no English equivalent for its embryological usage. 'Rudiment' or 'primordium' are the closest translations, but one can usually see a rudiment and a primordium. An anlage is an undelimited embryonic region prior to the first visible sign of differentiation.

The anlage of the pineal diverticulum is a dorsal median district of the neural tube at the level of the future diencephalon. The neural tube arises by the rolling up of a plate of ectoderm (the neural plate). In this event of development (neurulation) the margins of the plate, the neural folds (see Fig. 63), move together and fuse in the midline. Which neural fold carries the pineal anlage? Or do both contribute? The answer: Both folds carry prospective pineal-forming cells. So there are two pineal anlagen, each carried on the crest of a neural fold. As the folds unite, so do the two anlagen of the pineal diverticulum. This is not a unique developmental pattern. Certain other organs, such as heart and breastbone (sternum), also arise by fusion of two anlagen. The experimental embryologist can sometimes place a barrier (for example, a piece of foreign tissue) between them and cause the formation of two hearts or a divided sternum. Perhaps prevention of union of the neural folds in the diencephalic region might lead to the formation of paired pineal diverticula. So far as I know, this experiment has not been successfully conducted. However, Professor Albert Dalcq (1947) of the University of Brussels occasionally obtained two pineal bodies (epiphyses) as a result of rotating the upper (animal) hemisphere of early gastrulae of a European toad, *Discoglossus pictus.* The operation resulted in double embryos with varying degrees of incomplete brain formation. In some instances the neural folds were delayed in fusing or remained separated anteriorly, causing the formation of two pineal diverticula. Each differentiated into a pineal vesicle.

I cannot resist the temptation to bring death into this discussion of birth, because without the death of certain cells the normal development of a pineal diverticulum by fusion of its anlagen would not occur. When neural folds meet, nonsticky ectodermal cells are juxtaposed. Perhaps the closure of the neural tube cannot be completed, however, until cells along the line of apposition die, allowing the adhesive sides of neighboring cells to contact one another and become knitted together by cell junctions and by interdigitation. So death may be essential for life not only at levels of organisms and populations and at the biochemical level through cycling of building materials, but in the very midst of creation. Without cell death, when

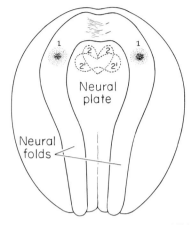

Fig. 63. Diagram of early amphibian embryo (mid-neurula stage), showing anlage of pineal diverticulum (1), and of lateral eyes at beginning of neurulation (2) and in early neurulation (2^1). Based upon Mangold (1931) and van de Kamer (1949); Emily E. Reid, delineator.

I was an embryo my fingers would not have been fashioned out of my paddlelike hands, and this essay would not have been written. Dr. Robert O. Kelley, formerly a doctoral student of mine, now on the faculty in anatomy at the University of New Mexico, has studied this specific problem (Kelley, 1970).

Why do embryonic cells die at the right time and at the right place? This is a profound question for which there is no answer at present. Is death initiated by events within the doomed cells, such as the release of digestive enzymes which destroy the cells (autolysis) or the elimination of critical organelles—mitochondria perhaps—by engulfment into vacuoles filled with digestive enzymes (autophagy)? Or are the cells attacked and eaten by their neighbors, a process which has been studied in the fruit-fly embryo by one of my students, Dr. Dianne Fristrom (1969)? Is it suicide or fratricide? We do not know. Another graduate student, Linda Mak, is at present seeking information on this point and on the subject under discussion—the possibility of cell death in neurulation.

Figure 63 shows diagrammatically the positions of the pineal anlagen (1) in an amphibian embryo at the time of formation of the neural folds as determined by vital staining experiments (van de Kamer, 1949). Anlagen are usually, if not always, larger than the organ rudiments which develop from them. They are areas or fields of cells which have the potentiality of forming specific embryonic structures. But not all cells in a district are actually involved, although each one *can* participate. The gradient in concentration of dots in the diagram is designed to show a gradient in developmental potency. Should the district be reduced, as by removal of part of it, the remaining cells could replace the missing ones and form a normal organ. The embryologists call this adjustment regulation. In the instance of the amphibian pineal diverticulum, regulation was demonstrated experimentally by Johan van de Kamer (1949) of Utrecht by removing the central parts of the anlagen. A pineal diverticulum formed nevertheless, although frequently it was small.

The anlagen of the lateral eyes (2′, Fig. 63) lie near the midline in the floor of the neural plate in the form of a dumbell-shaped area. Prior to neurulation the districts would have been a bilobed median region (2). In the instance of the lateral eyes, unlike heart and pineal diverticulum, there is at first a unified organ-forming area, which becomes subdivided into right and left anlagen. They separate and shift laterally owing to differential growth by cell multiplication between the two centers and by changing positions of individual cells. At the close of neurulation the lateral eye anlagen lie in the side walls of the future diencephalon. In Polyphemus and Sister One-Eye the anlagen failed to separate (see Preface).

Now, what establishes the pineal anlagen? Are they induced? I have pointed out earlier in defining induction that the neural tube is induced by underlying mesoderm. Accordingly, we may say that mesoderm underneath head ectoderm is the initiator of a chain of events that leads to the formation of the parietal-eye vesicle. Van de Kamer (1949) has performed instructive experiments on embryos of a salamander (*Amblystoma mexicanum*) and of the South African Clawed Toad (*Xenopus laevis*). He removed the pineal anlagen, transplanted them to other positions in the embryo, tested the inducing power of the underlying mesoderm by transplanting it to other sites, and so forth. Certain conclusions were possible from these experiments: The transplanted pineal anlagen cannot develop unless a diencephalon forms. Induction appears, therefore, to be limited in specificity. That is, the mesoderm evocates diencephalon but not pineal diverticulum alone. Once diencephalon is induced and begins to differentiate, the pineal primordium is evaginated.

To say that head mesoderm is the alpha of the development of a third eye is, of course, an incorrect or, at best, incomplete statement. Whence came the mesoderm? And where were the inducing substances formed and by what instructions? One is reminded of the nursery rhyme "This is the house that Jack built." Mesoderm originated from a band of cells near the equator of the earlier embryo (blastula), and their ancestry carries us back through cell divisions to the fertilized egg (zygote). The inducing substances were either already preformed and then made active and released by the mesoderm at the right time, or they were synthetized in the mesodermal cells just before neurulation. The latter alternative seems to be more likely. But in either event the instructions for making the particular chemical substances (probably proteins) that induced the neural tube and all of its derivatives must have come from the chromosomes or, more specifically, from the building codes of DNA carried by the chromosomes. And where did the chromosomes of mesoderm and zygote originate? They came into the embryo by way of the egg and the spermatozoon. Stop! It should be clear that this pursuit will not lead us to first causes.

Development of Lens

The lens of the third eye differs developmentally from that of the lateral eye in two fundamental features. We noted earlier that the lens of the parietal eye differentiates from the distal wall of the median optic vesicle (see Fig. 57). It is therefore a brain lens and consequently not homologous with the lens of the lateral eye, which arises from skin ectoderm. Second, whereas the cells of the embryonic lens of the lateral eye transform into curved crystalline fibers which collectively form a sphere or biconvex body, those of the parietal lens remain a palisade of columnar cells which at best is only slightly curved.

The nuclei of the lens cells migrate from the positions shown in Figure 26 toward the lumen of the eye, where they assume their permanent basal situation. The lower borders of the cells develop many microvilli and one cilium per cell, which project into the cavity of the eye like those from supportive cells (Fig. 62). Why should the undersurface of the lens be ciliated? Recall that these cells once lined the neural tube and such cells (ependymal) are ciliated. In the brain and spinal cord the beating of cilia moves the cerebrospinal fluid within the cavities of these organs. Perhaps the cilia of lens and supportive cells, assumed to be motile, stir the fluid within the lumen of the eye.

The cytoplasm of the embryonic lens cells appears to be highly active metabolically, judging by the large number of mitochondria and the organelles involved in the synthesis of cell products, namely, ribosomes and endoplasmic reticulum. One of these products is a fibrous material which accumulates in the distal (upper) part of the lens cells. As the volume of the secretion increases, the organelles of the cell just mentioned are crowded basally until the adult condition is reached. This fibrous material may be largely, if not entirely, specific lens proteins called crystallins.

Dr. David S. McDevitt (1972) of the University of Pennsylvania asked a very good question: Are the lens crystallins of the third eye the same as those in the lens of the lateral eye? By a very instructive experiment using a sophisticated technique called immunofluorescence he obtained the answer yes. The crystallins from the two types of eyes in the American Chameleon (*Anolis carolinensis*) appear to be of like chemical nature because the lens of the median eye reacts strongly with antibodies specific for lateral eye crystallins (Figs. 64, 65). Unless the two lenses were chemically alike, this reaction would not occur. Other proteins, such as those of the retina of the median eye, did not react with these antibodies.

The above experiment led McDevitt to a basic theoretical consideration about the synthesis of the median-eye crystallins. The genes carrying the code for the manufacture of the lens crystallins by the synthetic machinery in the cytoplasm can be activated (*turned on* is the expression used by the molecular biologist) in cells which differ in anatomical position, developmental and evolutionary history, and ultrastructural features. But what turns on the genes to

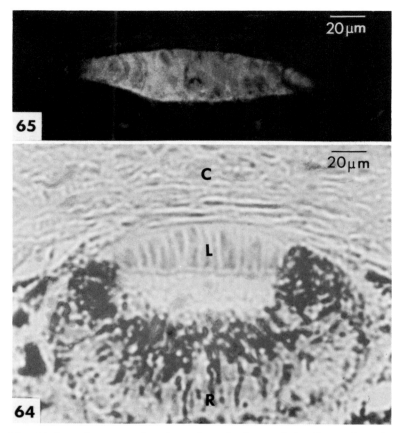

Fig. 64. LM of cross section through parietal eye of *Anolis carolinensis*. c, cornea; L, lens; R, retina. × 450.

Fig. 65. Darkfield fluorescence photomicrograph of cross section through parietal eye of *A. carolinensis*. Note, only lens fluoresces, showing binding of antibodies to lens proteins of lateral eye. × 450. Figs. 64 and 65 from McDevitt (1972); copyright 1972 by The American Association for the Advancement of Science. Courtesy of Dr. David S. McDevitt.

send out instructions to the cytoplasm, "Make lens crystallins"? Perhaps there is a lens activator (inductor) common to both median and lateral eyes. The sources of lens-inducing stimuli in the lateral eye are known: anterior entodermal and mesodermal cells underlying the ectodermal anlage of the lens (see Jacobson, 1963, and Mizuno,

1972) and the lateral optic vesicle (Spemann, 1938). But, as we have seen, the lens of the median eye arises from a part of the embryonic eye vesicle itself. I shall soon show that contact of the parietal vesicle with the skin is not essential for lens formation. In conclusion, we do not know what triggers lens differentiation in the parietal eye. The best help I can offer at this time is an old embryological cliché: the fate of a cell is a function of its position. There may be some factor in the embryonic microenvironment of the roof cells of the median optic vesicle which initiates the chain of molecular reactions leading to the secretion of lens crystallins. Perhaps this factor is the same as that inducing lens fiber formation in the lateral eye. My guess is that the triggers are different, but the effect is the same—the gun fires.

Origin of Parietal Nerve

A nerve is a bundle of nerve fibers, and a nerve fiber is an outgrowth of a nerve cell. In the embryo these presumptive nerve cells lie in or on the top of the neural tube. It was Ross Harrison, the foremost American experimental embryologist in the first part of this century, who brilliantly showed in the first use of cell culture that nerve fibers grow as slender cytoplasmic threads from embryonic nerve cells explanted into a culture medium, which in Harrison's experiment (1907) was a drop of lymph. Do the fibers of the parietal nerve arise in the brain or epiphysis and grow into the parietal optic vesicle, or vice versa? The answer to this question is not easily obtained from the embryo, because growing nerve fibers are difficult to identify and to trace. The literature shows conflicting opinions. So I attempted to solve the problem by studying degeneration in severed parietal nerves of adult lizards. It is well known that when a nerve is cut, the fibers on the side of the transection nearest the cell bodies, from which the fibers develop, do not degenerate, whereas those fibers beyond the incision degenerate because they are separated from the source of materials necessary for maintenance. Incidentally, recent research shows that this generalization does not apply to some invertebrates.

Severing the parietal nerve in *S. occidentalis* is an easy operation. A blue-bellied lizard is held with one hand under the dissecting microscope. Anesthesia is unnecessary. The large scale above the third eye (see Fig. 1) is removed but saved for later use, and an incision is made by a scalpel in the skin in front and to the sides of the eye. Then the skin is peeled back over the eye, exposing it and also the thin covering of the brain, the meninges, on the under surface of which lies the parietal nerve (see Fig. 25). One can make a neat transverse incision with a microknife through meninges and nerve a few millimeters behind the eye. Recall that the bony cranium is open in this region (pineal foramen). The microknife is fashioned from a sliver of razor blade edge soldered to a sewing needle, which is held by a chuck-type holder (Burch, 1942). The tip of the knife may be sharpened to a point on a powered grinding stone of fine quality. The incision made, the flap of skin is folded back into normal position, and the scale is added and sealed with a fast-drying solution of plastic (collodion).

After one to three days following surgery, animals were sacrificed and small segments of their parietal nerves anterior and posterior to the incision were removed, fixed, and sectioned. The ultrathin sections were examined in an electron microscope. Which segment of the nerve showed degeneration? The posterior one! The conclusion was inescapable: the parent cells of the nerve fibers lie in the eye and not in the brain (or epiphysis). The fibers of the nerve develop *from* the ganglion cells in the retina of the parietal eye just as the optic nerve fibers from the lateral eye are outgrowths of its ganglion cells (Eakin, 1964a).

Learning from Nature's Mistakes

Accidents in development (developmental anomalies) are often as instructive as the embryologist's experiments. Out of hundreds of blue-bellied lizards which Dr. Stebbins and I collected for our field and laboratory study (Stebbins and Eakin, 1958) and for subsequent investigations, we have encountered only two animals which appeared to have no third eyes. Upon microscopic examination, however, the eye in each of these instances was found attached to the tip of the epiphysis. I can only speculate on the cause of the incomplete subdivision of the pineal diverticulum at some embryonic stage;

perhaps there was a mechanical obstruction which prevented the "migration" of the parietal vesicle to its normal position. In some lizards (see Schmidt, 1909) the parietal eye and epiphysis are very closely associated normally. The latter is a long tube which extends upward and forward to within a few tenths of a millimeter of the parietal eye.

One of our two unusual specimens is shown in Figure 66. The out-of-place (ectopic) eye is fully differentiated into lens, retina, and capsule. The retina contains normal sensory, supportive, and ganglion cells typically arranged, except for irregularities at the junction between eye and epiphysis. The parietal and epiphysial lumens are not continuous, but their capsules are smoothly fused. Axons from the eye appear to emerge from the ventral surface of the retina and to pass directly into the epiphysis. The eye lies below the roof of the cranium (CR) and is attached to the meninges of the brain. Farther forward the cranium is perforated by a normal parietal foramen, minus its usual occupant; but the skin above it is not a transparent cornea. Instead, it is like the integument in general: nontransparent, thick, and containing pigmented cells (Eakin, 1964a).

Certain inferences can be drawn from this experiment of nature. First, the development of the eye is not dependent upon the attainment of its normal position above the cerebrum, outside the meninges, and in intimate association with the skin. Second, the parietal eye appears to be a self-differentiating organ, to use an old-fashioned embryological expression. Once the anterior part of the pineal diverticulum has been determined (that is, its course of differentiation irreversibly programed at the biochemical level), it proceeds to form a normal eye so far as is possible in its abnormal position. To state it differently, there is no smooth transition of one organ into the other, as one would expect if they possessed plasticity and regulatory capability in the early embryo. Finally, the differentiation of the cornea appears to be dependent upon the inductive action of the parietal vesicle or perhaps more specifically the lens of the third eye. In the development of the vertebrate lateral eye the lens provides the stimulus for the differentiation of the skin into a clear cornea (see Mangold, 1931).

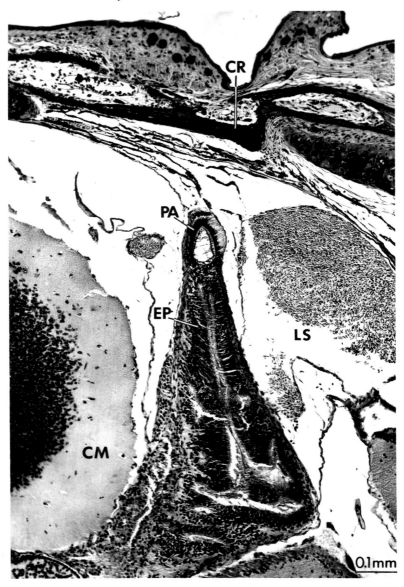

Fig. 66. Lм of median longitudinal (sagittal) section through head of
S. occidentalis possessing abnormal parietal eye (PA) attached to tip
of epiphysis (EP). CM, cerebrum of brain; CR, bony cranium; LS, large
blood vessel (longitudinal sinus). × 112. Eakin, Stebbins, and Ortman,
from Eakin (1964*a*).

The above account of the developmental history of third eyes has answered the questions posed at the beginning, but it has raised others which cannot be solved at this time. With a modest background of information on the evolution, structure, and embryonic origin of the vertebrate median eye and its parts, we are now ready to consider the all-important topic: its function.

5

Function

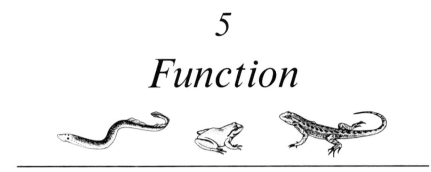

For the climax and finale of my play all of the characters are on the stage ready to speak to the questions "what good is a third eye?" "does it really function?" and "if so, how?" It is clear from the record that almost every biologist who has studied a third eye, from Stieda, Leydig, and Studnička to the last character in this cast, has endeavored to direct some light on its physiological role. Ideas and suggestions have not been wanting, as a brief review of the literature will disclose. Did I hear the reader protest, or was it my imagination? I thought that I heard: "Why bother with ancient history? There is no point in exhuming dead notions and foolish hypotheses. There has already been too much history in this play—evolutionary history, developmental history, anatomical history, and now . . . ?"

As author and a member of the cast, I have a right to say a few lines. I am a firm believer in history, history of any kind. And I protest the arrogance of many scientists who dismiss it as being without much value. History in science gives us perspective, a fuller understanding of the subject under study, insight into pitfalls and difficulties in research on a given problem, inspiration from our predecessors and their work—often heroic—and lastly a camaraderie among scientists transcending separation by race, culture, and time.

In preparing this book I have been illuminated, astonished, excited by reading the works of biologists who have studied vertebrate pineals in the last century. The pages of some of their works are yellowed with age, an occasional page is still uncut, others are underlined by pencil and stained with coffee—evidence of much use; in all the words and illustrations are rich with the observations and the thoughts of dedicated men and women. Thanks to the wisdom of some of my professors, notably Charles Atwood Kofoid, the biology library at Berkeley is remarkably complete in these works. The administration of the university was persuaded to build a magnificent treasury of knowledge. Kofoid himself collected and donated to the biology library over 70,000 pamphlets and 61,000 volumes, many of them first editions of zoological classics. And Willis Linn Jepson made a munificent gift of botanical works. Hail, noble scholars and bibliophiles!

A Hundred and One Theories

A new theory each year for a century? Well, not really, but there have been several on the function of the third eye.

1. NO FUNCTION.

A few biologists, especially those in the late 1800s, who observed third eyes of vertebrates and contemplated their role, came to the conclusion that pineal and parietal eyes are without function. They are only useless vestiges of ancient visual organs. Simple experiments involving illumination or shading of parietal eyes of lizards gave no indication of function. Parietal eyes and frontal organs are lacking altogether in many reptiles and amphibians; consequently, third eyes are nonessential. Many students have been unable to find a nerve leading from these organs, even in recent times (Steyn, 1957; Roth and Braun, 1958). I am in correspondence now with a young man who is having difficulty in identifying the parietal nerve in a group of lizards. In fact, I am embarrassed to recall that Dr. Stebbins and I overlooked that nerve in *Sceloporus* at first, owing to its obscurity in the transverse sections we were using. We corrected our error (Eakin and Stebbins, 1959), however, and demonstrated its presence in eight other species of lizards. Meanwhile, electron microscopy (Eakin and Westfall, 1959, 1960) proved that the nerve was indeed a bundle of many axons from the ganglion cells.

The most negative position on the question of function of the reptilian third eye in relatively recent times is that of Roth and Braun (1958), who were unable to demonstrate responsiveness to light or temperature by the parietal eye of the Slow Worm *Anguis fragilis*. They concluded, therefore, that the organ was rudimentary and, I assume, without function. At this time (1972) with the new information on fine structure and neurological activity of third eyes (see below), I doubt that anyone believes them to be functionless.

2. LOOKOUT FOR THE DEVIL.

But what do third eyes do? I shall proceed from the ridiculous (this hypothesis) to the sublime (our theory). Anyone discussing the raison d'être of any part of the pineal complex is expected to mention, I suppose, the notion of the seventeenth-century French philosopher René Descartes that the epiphysis is the seat of the soul. This proposition appeared in his book *De homine* ('On Man'), which was published posthumously in Latin in 1662 and in French in 1664. A new English translation appeared in 1972. Had man a third eye, it would have been logical for Descartes to suggest that it served as a lookout for the devil, to warn the soul of his presence. But man has no third eye, and animals with the eye have no soul, according to Descartes, so this hypothesis is untenable.

3. THERMORECEPTORAL FUNCTION.

The hypothesis that the parietal eye of lizards was a temperature-sensitive organ was first suggested by Rabl-Rückhard (1886). He believed that the eye might serve to warn its bearer against over-exposure to radiation of high intensity. Along the same line, Willem Steyn (1961) theorized that a third eye may have had survival value in the first terrestrial vertebrates by alerting them to desiccation. Nowikoff (1910) rejected the idea of thermoreceptivity because some tropical reptiles, such as crocodiles, do not posses the third eye and because the sensory cells of the parietal eye do not contain pigment granules (assumed to be necessary for the absorption of heat), whereas pigment is present in the supportive cells. To Nowi-koff's arguments I add further objections to the hypothesis of tem-perature sensitivity. In the first place, the fine structure of thermore-ceptors, in the few instances studied, is unlike that of photoreceptors. The receptoral apparatus of the thermal-sensitive pit organ of vipers, for example, consists of a mass of branchlets of nerve fibers (Bleich-mar and De Robertis, 1962; Terashima, Goris, and Katsuki, 1970). In insects thermoreceptors are probably hairlike sensilla on antennae and legs or multidendritic endings in thin areas of cuticle (Slifer, 1953). Second, thermal sensitivity is widespread over the skin of a lizard. I found in experiments with blinded *Sceloporus* (lateral eyes removed) that a bright spot of light, whose heat I could detect with the back of my hand, elicited responses from the lizard when the beam was directed upon any dorsal area of the body. I did not test the animal's ventral surface. Roth and Braun (1958) reported similar findings on blinded *Anguis fragilis*.

4. PRODUCTION OF ANTIRACHITIC (VITAMIN D) SUBSTANCES.

Steyn (1959b) put forth another novel suggestion that the pigmented cells of the parietal eyes of lizards "are migratory and may transport antirachitic substances formed in the organ while the animal suns itself, out of the organ's retina during darkness at night or when the animal is in the shade." I believe that the pigmented cells which Steyn observed in the lumen of the parietal eye of three species of South African lizards are not pigmented cells from the retina but macrophages. And I speculate that the pigmented cells which he observed external to the eye and believed to be outward migrating cells are also macrophages. I too have observed pigmented cells in the vicinity of the third eye of *Sceloporus* which look like mac-rophages to me. I cannot disprove, however, that these cells are carrying vitamin D, as postulated by Steyn.

5. INHIBITOR OF SEXUAL ACTIVITY.

Having mentioned the divine above, perhaps I should give equal time to the carnal. Clausen and Poris (1937) of the American

Museum of Natural History conducted an experimental study of testicular activity in the American Chameleon *Anolis carolinensis* with and without the parietal eye. They found that obliteration of the organ resulted in a tendency toward acceleration of sperm production. They suggested that the eye "may act as an inhibitor of testicular activation or that an internal secretion is liberated by the pineal eye which in turn results, either directly or indirectly, in the production of inhibiting influences toward sexual stimulation." Since this proposed function rests upon the eye's sensitivity to light, the hypothesis will be considered later under Item 7, photoreceptoral function.

6. SECRETORY FUNCTION.

We have noted earlier that Stieda (1865), who first discovered the frontal organ in amphibians, thought that it was a gland. Holmgren (1918) and Oksche (1952) advanced this notion by careful cytological studies. They demonstrated a variable picture in the structure and staining characteristics of the sensory processes. Holmgren (1918) postulated a cyclical degeneration and regeneration in the outer segments of the frontal organ of a frog, *Rana temporaria*. He speculated further that there was a flow of secretion from the nucleus to the outer segment through that part of the sensory cell called an ellipsoid. Refinements were added to this picture by Oksche (1952), who then doubted that the frontal organ had a sensory function. The discovery of conelike or rodlike outer segments by electron microscopy, however, revived the hypothesis that the frontal organ was a photoreceptor (see below).

Where do we stand, then, on the notion that the stirnorgan is secretory? Could it and other third eyes be both sensory and secretory? We have noted that there is an apparent sloughing of the outer segments in some third eyes, particularly in the pineal vesicle of lampreys and in the amphibian frontal organ. Stacks and whorls of disks accumulate in the cavities of these organs. Kelly (1962) has pointed out that, whereas this exfoliation of the outer segments might be considered a form of secretion, Holmgren's ideas of cyclical degeneration and regeneration are more applicable. In the parietal eye of lizards, however, one does not see so many cast-off disks, perhaps because macrophages keep the lumen relatively free of debris or because the outer segments are more stable. If it were not for the phagocytic activity of macrophages in parietal eyes and the pigmented epithelium in lateral eyes, cast-off disks of outer segments might amass as in the pineal vesicles of lamprey and frog, where a scavenging and recycling mechanism may be less well developed. Regarding photoreceptive pineal structures of lower vertebrates, Kelly (1962) concluded: "ultrastructural evidence produced to date does not indicate much in the way of secretory activity—at least not in the usual sense of neuro-, exo-, or endocrine secretion. . . . if secretion is occurring it is on a subtle basis, perhaps subsidiary to photoreceptive processes." Considering, however, the increasing evidence of secretory activity in sensory cells of the epiphysis (see discussions by Professors Ariëns Kappers and Andreas Oksche in a recent symposium volume edited by Wolstenholme and Knight, 1971) and considering the similarity of third-eye receptors to those in the epiphysis, it appears that this hypothesis is still viable.

7. PHOTORECEPTORAL FUNCTION.

Early investigators of the third eye in lizards naturally attributed a photosensory role to that organ because of its anatomical similarity to lateral eyes (see Studnička, 1905). They recognized, however, the improbability that the eye could form a visual image on its retina because of inadequacies of its optical apparatus. The argument for light-sensitivity was succinctly summarized by Nowikoff (1907, 1910): The entire structure of the organ shows an unmistakable adaptation for receiving light. One can scarcely conclude that the parietal eye is rudimentary if one considers the highly differentiated state of the retina with three cell types, one of which possesses sensory processes, the transparency of cornea and lens, and the presence of a nerve connecting the organ to the brain. This hypothesis of a photoreceptoral role received further support from our discovery of the conelike (or rodlike) ultrastructure of the retinal processes in the third eyes of a lizard, a frog, and a lamprey. But physiological evidence was needed.

Many investigators had conducted simple experiments, such as sudden illumination or shading of the third eye (for example,

Nowikoff, 1910; Dendy, 1911), to no avail so far as eliciting any response from the animal went. Unconvinced by the failures of my predecessors, I, too, tried photosensitivity tests on the parietal eye of blue-bellies from which I had removed the lateral eyes. I reasoned that one could not successfully test the light-responsivenes of the third eye of a lizard without first eliminating the dominant photoreceptors of the animal. I learned to perform ophthalmectomy with minimal hemorrhage and to nurture the blinded Scelops for many weeks by feeding them on alternate days with small capsules filled with food. The mouth was forced open and held in that position while a loaded capsule, made slippery with glycerine, was pushed into the stomach with a smooth probe. The blinded Scelops made wonderful pets, which children loved because they would not bite or run away. But, despite much patient study and experimentation, I was unable to obtain consistent behavioral responses to light of varying wavelength and intensity directed upon the parietal eye. I have not previously recorded these efforts.

More productive were the field and laboratory studies which Dr. Stebbins and I conducted from 1955 to 1957 and published in 1958. These will be reviewed shortly. Although our findings strongly supported the theory of the light-sensitivity of the parietal eye of *Sceloporus* (hypothesis had advanced to theory!) we could not assert it as a fact. We could not demonstrate responsivity to light in an individual lizard.

An Effort to Demonstrate a Photopigment.

I undertook another line of attack. I enlisted the collaboration of a friend in zoology on our Los Angeles campus, Professor Frederick Crescitelli, in an effort to demonstrate a light-sensitive chemical (photopigment) in the parietal eye of *S. occidentalis*. Would he make a laboratory test (spectrophotometry) if I provided the material? Yes, he would. So I began stockpiling third eyes from blue-bellies. I remember one weekend of hard collecting by my family which yielded enough Scelops to keep me busy for several days extirpating dark-adapted third eyes under dim red illumination and storing them in a frozen state. My bank finally totaled 110 eyes. I sent them to Fred Crescitelli with high hopes, but the result was negative: "No demonstrable photopigment in the extract. Sample probably too small." Even the thought of trying to double the stalking, noosing, and decapitating of the blue-bellies and tediously removing their third eyes under a dissecting microscope in a dark room was too much. Moreover, the slaughter of 110 of these freedom-loving creatures to obtain a few micrograms of tissue, even in the cause of science, had been a burden on my conscience. My feelings of guilt were partly assuaged by the use of the bodies of the animals by another biologist (Dr. John Davis of our Museum of Vertebrate Zoology) for a study of food preferences. To this day a photopigment has not been isolated from any third eye or, indeed, from the lateral eye of any diurnal lizard.

Vitamin A Deficiency.

I then undertook a still different approach, a nutritional study. It had been known for a number of years that vitamin A deficiency causes anatomical degeneration in the retina. Then John Dowling and Nobel laureate George Wald (1958, 1960) made the stunning discovery that weanling rats maintained on a vitamin-A–free diet became night-blind after five months. Their visual threshold corresponded to the loss of 96 to 98 percent of the photopigment from their eyes. And Dowling and Gibbons (1961) demonstrated that vitamin A deficiency causes degeneration in the outer segments of retinal rods in rats. The disks became swollen and then fragmented into vesicles, and by the end of eight months of the malnutrition only remnants of the outer segments could be observed. In the fall of 1960 I began an experiment on a group of fence lizards in which the animals were sustained solely on gelatin capsules filled with a diet lacking vitamin A. The experiment was terminated a year later, and their lateral and median eyes were prepared for electron microscopy. I obtained results similar to those of Dowling and Gibbons —namely, vesicular degeneration in the outer segments of cones of the lateral eye of *Sceloporus* (rods are absent in diurnal lizards) and of the sensory processes of the parietal eye (Fig. 67).

The reader will recall that vitamin A (actually the aldehyde of the vitamin or retinaldehyde) is the light-sensitive part of a photopigment. Without the vitamin an eye cannot make photopigments, and the animal becomes blind. And, for some as yet unexplained reason, the disks of the outer segments degenerate. Here, then, was further

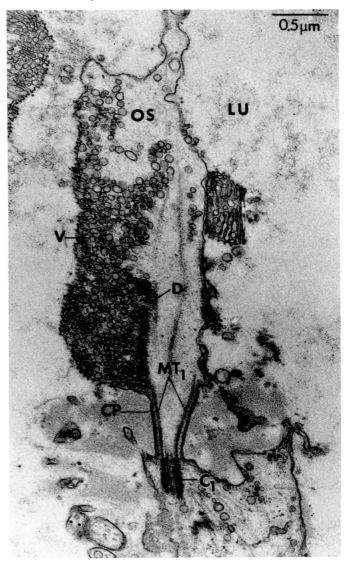

Fig. 67. Em of longitudinal section through ciliary photoreceptor in parietal eye of *S. occidentalis* deficient in vitamin A. c_1,
distal centriole (kinetosome); CP, connecting piece; D, remnants of disks; LU, lumen of eye; MT_1, microtubules (axoneme)
of cilium; OS, outer segment; V, vesicles resulting from breakdown of disks. × 27,000. Eakin and Westfall, from Eakin
(1964*b*).

evidence of the light-sensitivity of a parietal eye: it exhibited the same type of degeneration owing to vitamin A deficiency as the lateral eyes. By the time I published this investigation (Eakin, 1964*b*) the electrical studies, soon to be discussed, had established the photoreceptoral function of third eyes.

Stirnorganectomy.

While waiting for the vitamin A experiment on *Sceloporus* to run its course, I began a study of the frontal organ, or stirnorgan, in tadpoles of *Hyla regilla*. Jane Westfall and I discovered that its sensory processes exhibited ciliary outer segments like those in the reptilian parietal eye. I promptly conducted some experiments on larvae from which I removed the frontal organ by surgery (stirnorganectomy). The results of both the electron microscopy and extirpation experiments were published together (Eakin, 1961). I regret that I did not include Jane Westfall, then a research assistant, as a coauthor; she cut the ultrathin sections and made the micrographs. I hasten to add, however, that I am not an armchair biologist. I was and am a practicing electron microscopist.

The stirnorgan is clearly visible through the transparent epidermis in young tadpoles of *Hyla*, and it is easily removed through an incision in the skin by means of microknife and microscissors fashioned from strips of razor blade (Eakin and Westfall, 1965). I looked for a disturbance in the control of the animal's pigmentation. Bagnara (1960) had just demonstrated that the blanching reaction of the body skin, commonly exhibited by amphibian larvae when placed in the dark, was lost upon destruction of the epiphysis in tadpoles of the South African Clawed Toad *Xenopus laevis*. The blanching reaction is produced chiefly by the concentration of melanin pigment near the nuclei of the melanophores in the skin (see Fig. 68), whereas in the unblanched animal the pigment is dispersed into the many cytoplasmic processes of the melanophores (see Fig. 69). Incidentally, the above illustrations of aggregated and dispersed melanin are taken from another type of study by one of my doctoral students, William T. Driscoll, now a dean at the University of Denver, and me. They serve adequately, however, to demonstrate the two states of melanin distribution.

I compared my stirnorganectomized tadpoles with control animals

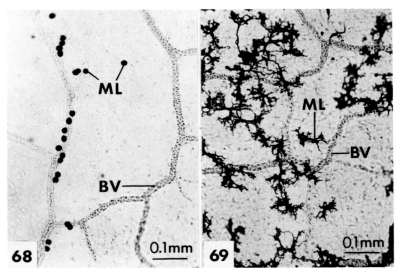

Figs. 68 and 69. Melanophores (ML) with pigment concentrated and dispersed in, respectively, the skin of albino (Fig. 68) and the skin of normal (Fig. 69) tadpoles of *H. regilla*. BV, blood vessel containing corpuscles. × 86. From Driscoll and Eakin (1955).

(sibling tadpoles, in which I made an incision in the skin to one side of the frontal organ). A significant difference between the coloration of experimental and control animals was not manifest, however, until I removed the lateral eyes from both groups. Then the body-blanching reaction was reduced or disappeared altogether in most of the experimentals, whereas most of the controls continued to blanch when placed in the dark. In many of those controls which did not show the reaction over the body, there was a distinct contraction of the melanophores in the vicinity of the frontal organ.

From the above experiment I drew the conclusion that the stirn-organ was demonstrably photosensitive. Light apparently inhibits the frontal organ from sending neural impulses to the epiphysis, but in the absence of light that inhibition is removed. Impulses carried in the parietal nerve presumably stimulate the epiphysis to release a hormone which causes the "contraction" of dermal melanophores and a consequent blanching of the animal. I postulated that the positive reaction in some of the experimental larvae might be due to the presence of photoreceptors in the epiphysis. No explanation was advanced at that time, however, for the absence of the blanching reaction in a few controls despite intact frontal organs. On the basis of further work of Bagnara (1963, 1964), I now suggest that those controls had sufficient circulating melanophore-stimulating hormone (MSH) from the pituitary gland to counteract the pineal hormone (melatonin, see Lerner et al., 1958). An excellent history of studies on the relation of the epiphysis to pigmentation is given by Bagnara and Hadley (1970).

I should cite the study of Stebbins, Steyn, and Peers (1960) on the effects of stirnorganectomy in tadpoles of an African frog, *Pyxicephalus delalandi*. There were no differences between experimental and control larvae with respect to coloration of the animals, whether in the dark or in the light. Control animals had received a sham operation; that is, they were subjected to surgical trauma by an incision in the skin to one side of the frontal organ. Moreover, no difference between the two types was noted in regard to locomotor activity, rate of development, or exposure to sunlight. I wonder, however, whether the removal of the lateral eyes from the tadpoles of both groups would have changed the results of the experiment.

Light- and Dark-adaptation.

I next endeavored to demonstrate some significant difference between the parietal eyes of *S. occidentalis* and of the Side-blotched Lizard *Uta stansburiana* maintained in total darkness for varying periods of time and the third eyes of comparable animals subjected to continuous illumination with a bright light for equal lengths of time. I confirmed the observation of Nowikoff (1907, 1910) that there is a shift in pigment in the supportive cells of *Lacerta agilis* and *Anguis fragilis* toward the back of the retina in dark-adapted lizards and toward the lumen of the eye in light-adapted specimens. Although the movement of the pigment was not so dramatic as that described by Nowikoff, it demonstrated light-sensitivity in the parietal eyes studied. I do not know whether the photic stimulus was received directly by the supportive cells or first by the sensory elements which then transmitted an excitation to the pigment-bearing cells. My observations were recorded in a paper by Eakin, Quay, and Westfall (1961). Professor Wilbur Quay needs no introduction to pinealogists, as he is one of the leading authorities on avian and mammalian pineals. He brought to our studies on the third eyes of lower vertebrates an expertise in cytochemical methods.

In the above-mentioned paper we reported another difference between light- and dark-adapted parietal eyes. Glycogen, a complex carbohydrate important as a source of energy, was more abundant in the latter than in the former. The relative amounts of the compound were judged subjectively by comparing the reactions of the two types of eyes to a stain which generally reveals carbohydrates (periodic acid-Schiff reaction). Stores of glycogen are most common in the supranuclear regions of the sensory cells of *Sceloporus*, in the lens, and in the cavity of the parietal eye. Our observations that light-adapted eyes contained less glycogen than dark-adapted ones again suggested the photosensitivity of the third eye.

Parietal Eyes in Burrowing Lizards.

I have had the pleasure of correspondence with a graduate student at the University of Pittsburgh, G. Craig Gundy, who recently studied the third eye in members of the family Scincidae, which includes both burrowing and diurnal forms. At one end of the scale is *Feylinia currori*, which is limbless and burrowing; it possesses no parietal foramen, although there is a slight thinning of the parietal bone; and the parietal eye is said to be degenerate. At the other end of the range is the diurnal skink, with well-developed limbs, a large parietal foramen, and an excellent third eye (Gundy and Ralph, 1971). Gundy (1972) concludes that "a burrowing life style is correlated with closure of the parietal foramen" and "parietal eye development is correlated with the relative amount of light to which the animal is normally exposed." I assume that these statements are to be interpreted in the sense of evolution of the parietal eye in skinks.

As the following two sections are by necessity somewhat technical, the general reader may wish to proceed to the topic "Dosimeter of Solar Radiation."

Neurophysiological Studies (Reptilian).

The recording of an electrical response from an organ or its nerve when the organ is illuminated is generally considered indubitable proof of its light-sensitivity. Neither Dr. Stebbins nor I possessed the equipment or experience to conduct neurophysiological investigations on the third eye of *Sceloporus*. We obtained, however, the collaboration of a young neurophysiologist, Dr. Duco Hamasaki, in our school of optometry through our good friend and inspiring colleague Gordon Lynn Walls. We began a series of experiments on *Sceloporus* early in 1961. Our first efforts were unsuccessful. Before we could perfect our tehnique, William H. Miller of the Rockefeller Institute and Myron L. Wolbarsht of the Naval Medical Research Institute (both have made professional moves subsequently) published a short paper in *Science* describing and figuring the first electrical recording (electroretinogram, or ERG) from the retina of a reptilian third eye. With their kind permission I am privileged to reproduce two of their recordings (Fig. 70) from the parietal eye of the American Chameleon *Anolis carolinensis*. Incidentally, *Anolis* and its third eye made the cover of the issue of *Science* bearing the article (January 26, 1962).

Miller and Wolbarsht found that one-tenth of a second after illumination of a parietal eye the glass electrode on the retina became negative with respect to the other electrode placed in the mouth of the anole (in Fig. 70A "negative" is up). Throughout illumination the negative potential was sustained, but upon turning the light off the potential returned to the resting level. Figure 70B shows the vigorous discharge of impulses (on-response) recorded by a metal electrode on the retina and another burst of activity (off-response) when the light was discontinued. The duration of illumination (four seconds in this experiment) is shown by the line below the trace of activity.

No further recording was conducted on the reptilian parietal eye until 1968, when Professor Eberhard Dodt of the Max Planck Institute in Bad Nauheim, Germany, and his colleagues turned their electrodes from the amphibian frontal organ to the third eye of a lizard, *Lacerta sicula*. They considerably advanced the analysis of nervous activity of a parietal eye beyond the findings of Miller and Wolbarsht.

Dodt and Scherer (1968*a*, *b*) obtained slow, graded, positive potentials (Fig. 71A), which were associated with inhibition of nerve impulses. They resembled the response (specifically, the b-wave of the ERG) from the lizard's lateral eye (Fig. 71B), except for the re-

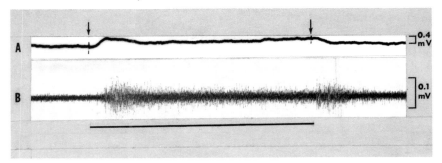

Fig. 70. First electroretinogram from parietal eye. Recorded from *A. carolinensis.* Responses to illumination: (A) d–c recording. (B) a–c recording. Arrows indicate artifacts resulting from shutter operation. For both records heavy line under B indicates presence of stimulus. Positive potential at recording electrodes is down. From Miller and Wolbarsht (1962); copyright 1962 by The American Association for the Advancement of Science. Courtesy of Dr. Myron L. Wolbarsht.

versal of electrical polarity. These investigators attributed this difference in electrical polarity to the difference in structural polarity. The receptors extended forward in the parietal eye, backward in the lateral eye. The response of the parietal eye was slower than that of the paired eyes, and it required an illuminance one thousand times that needed to elicit a response from the lateral eye. The last difference was explained by Dodt and Scherer as the result of the poorer light-gathering power of the cornea and lens (dioptric apparatus) of the median eye and by its simpler neurological organization. The parietal eye has a two-cell chain of conductors (receptor cell-ganglion cell), whereas the lateral eye enjoys a three-cell pathway (receptor cell-bipolar neurone-ganglion cell). The pooling of impulses (summation) is probably greater in the latter than in the former. And there may be other contributing factors inherent in the more complex organization of the lateral eye compared with that of the median eye (for example, presence and absence, respectively, of horizontal and amacrine cells).

A further difference of importance between the electrical records from parietal eye and those from lateral eyes relates to responsiveness to light of varying wavelength. The responses noted above (Fig. 71A, B) were elicited by violet light (428 nm). If green (530 nm) light is used, the polarity of the response of the median eye is reversed (Fig. 71C), and the response is a negative potential change associated with an increase in neural activity (excitation). There is no significant change, however, in the ERG of the lateral eye (Fig. 71D). The parietal eye of the lizard is color-sensitive! Its sensitivity peaks at about 450 nm and again at 520 nm, in the blue and green, respectively, whereas that of the lateral eye shows one peak, at 560 nm (as expected from an all-cone retina). In addition to the slow, graded responses just discussed, Dodt and Scherer (1968*a*, *b*) obtained fast nervous impulses, as did Miller and Wolbarsht (1962). These authors (Dodt and Scherer, 1968*a*) speculate that the slow responses reflect activity of structures near the photoreceptors, whereas the fast ones represent discharges from the ganglion cells of the eye.

Simultaneously with the studies in Germany on *Lacerta*, Duco Hamasaki (1968) made recordings from the third eye of the Green Iguana (*Iguana iguana*) at the University of Miami school of medicine. He found that the response of the eye to white light (achromatic stimuli) consisted of two components: (1) a positive on-response and a negative off-response and (2) a negative on-response and no response at the end of illumination. The two components differed in several features. Hamasaki concluded that the parietal eye of the iguana has physiological characteristics which are more like those of the lateral eyes of nocturnal reptiles, such as geckos and caimans, than like those of the iguana's lateral eyes. In a second study Hamasaki (1969*a*) determined the sensitivity of the third eye of the Green Iguana to light of different wavelengths. His results agreed with those of Dodt and Scherer with respect to recordings from the parietal eye (they did not agree on the spectral sensitivity of the lateral eyes). Hamasaki (1969*b*), contrary to Dodt and Scherer (1968*a*), believed that the slow, graded responses of a reptilian third eye originated in the ganglion cells. He conjectured further: "Stimulation of the blue-sensitive photoreceptors elicits the positive component from the ganglion cells and stimulation of the green-sensitive photoreceptors the negative component."

For further features of the neurophysiological activity in the parietal eye of lizards the reader is referred to the studies cited above

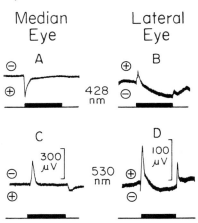

Fig. 71. Graded responses to light of different wavelengths by parietal and lateral eyes of *Lacerta sicula*. Horizontal black bars indicate duration of stimuli. Simplified from Dodt and Scherer (1968); Emily E. Reid, delineator.

and to a chapter by Professor Dodt, which I have not had the pleasure of seeing, expected soon in volume 7, part 3 of *Handbook of Sensory Physiology* (1973).

Neurophysiological Studies (Amphibian).

The first report on electrical activity in a third eye was a note in 1961 by Ewald Heerd and Eberhard Dodt on responses to illumination by the frontal organ of *Rana temporaria*. A more extensive report was published by Dodt and Heerd the following year (1962). Apparently these authors did not know at that time about our electron microscopical studies on the frontal organ of *Hyla regilla* and the parietal eye of *Sceloporus occidentalis*. By electrical recording from the pineal nerve (see Fig. 72A) they made an elegant analysis of the light-sensitivity of the stirnorgan. This important paper plus subsequent ones by Dodt and his collaborators (see Dodt, 1973) are the foundation of our present knowledge of the neurophysiology of amphibian pineal organs.

It was shown by the German workers that light is the only stimulus which changes the activity in the frontal or pineal nerve of adult

Rana temporaria (or *R. esculenta*); infrared, mechanical, and chemical stimuli are ineffective. The frontal organ is sensitive to a broad range of radiation from the ultraviolet to the red end of the visible spectrum (from 321 to 727 nm in wavelength). The responses are from two systems of the eye (that is, two groups of cells)—achromatic and chromatic. The two systems differ in the kind of response they make to light. The former reacts "to qualitatively different stimuli with the same unspecific response," and the latter exhibits "consistent differences in responses to light stimuli of different wavelengths" (Dodt and Heerd, 1962). The achromatic system is purely inhibitory with all wavelengths and is followed by vigorous off-responses (Fig. 72B); maximal sensitivity is highest at about 560 to 580 nm; in some animals there is a secondary peak at 380 nm. The chromatic response, on the other hand, has two components: (1) medium and long wavelengths (blue-green to red, 434 to 673 nm) elicit excitatory responses (Fig. 72C); maximal sensitivity is about 515 nm. (2) Short wavelengths (ultraviolet to blue; 321 to 448 nm) produce inhibition of the normal spontaneous activity (Fig. 72D); maximal sensitivity lies at 355 nm. The excitatory responses were recorded after first conditioning the organ with ultraviolet radiation, the inhibitory ones after conditioning with blue-free light.

The transition from a state of inhibition to excitation did not occur in a single step. Dodt and Heerd (1962) speculated that the photosensory mechanism probably has a simple photochemical basis: the inhibitory responses may be mediated by absorption of light within the α band (355 λ max) and the excitatory responses by absorption of light within the β band (515 λ max) of the same photopigment, namely, rhodopsin. The receptive part of the photopigment is probably vitamin A_1 aldehyde (retinaldehyde).

Other differences between chromatic and achromatic responses have been noted by Dodt and his associates. There is no change in threshold of the chromatic response after exposure to white light; the threshold of the achromatic response, however, is greatly modified by light- or dark-adaptation. It is difficult to separate the achromatic from chromatic responses in the amphibian frontal nerve, which contains a mixture of medullated and nonmedullated fibers (Oksche and von Harnack, 1962). Dodt and Heerd (1962) achieved this, however, by subjecting the third eye to ultraviolet radiation of

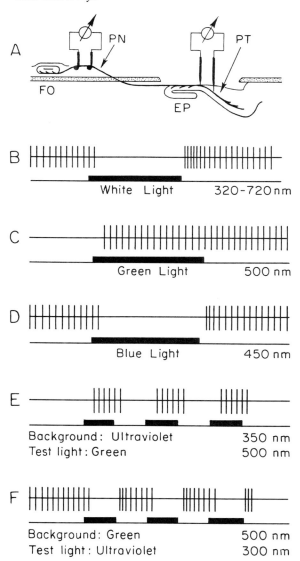

suitable intensity and duration to inhibit the chromatic responses, leaving the achromatic responses unaffected. The impulses responsible for the chromatic response appear to be carried by both medullated and nonmedullated nerve fibers in the frontal nerve, whereas those for the achromatic response are conducted by medullated axons only.

The activity of the frontal nerve differs from that of vertebrate optic nerves in at least one primary respect. The stirnorgan responds to long wavelengths by sustained excitation; conversely, short wavelengths (for example, ultraviolet) elicit sustained inhibition. In both instances the response may be continued for minutes after the cessation of the stimulus and even after reillumination with the same wavelength. But sustained excitation can be broken by exposure of the stirnorgan to short wavelengths and, conversely, sustained inhibition by illumination with long wavelengths. If, for example, the frontal organ is given a continuous background illumination of weak ultraviolet radiation (350 nm) and is periodically exposed to brief tests of strong green light (500 nm), the eye responds with short bursts of nervous impulses (Fig. 72E). On the other hand, background illumination with green light, which produces continuous excitation, and tests with ultraviolet give periods of no response (inhibition) (Fig. 72F). The responses, excitation or inhibition, always follow shortly after onset of the test light (lag) and continue briefly after the test light is extinguished.

Dodt, Ueck, and Oksche (1971) have speculated that the achromatic response may be the result of an inhibitory action on the ganglion cells by receptors containing one or two photopigments. In the chromatic response, on the other hand, both excitatory and inhibitory actions interact, depending on the quality of the stimulating light. Perhaps sensory cells with different photopigments synapse on the same ganglion cell. The ultraviolet-blue–absorbing cell may

---

Fig. 72. Responses of frontal organ of *Rana esculenta.* (A) Position of electrodes for recording from parietal (pineal) nerve (PN) which leads from frontal organ (FO), or from pineal tract (PT) which leads from epiphysis (EP). To place electrodes on latter, an opening was made in bony cranium, represented by stippled layer. (B) Response to white light (achromatic). (C–F) Chromatic responses to light of different wavelengths. Duration of test stimuli shown by horizontal black bars. A, C, and D from Dodt (1968); B, E, and F from Dodt, Ueck, and Oksche (1971); Emily E. Reid, delineator.

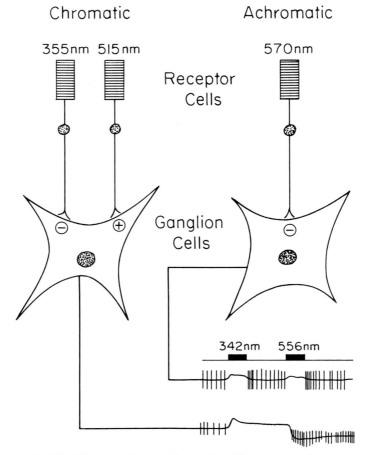

Fig. 73. Diagram of probable relationship between photoreceptors and ganglion cells in frontal organ of frogs. Chromatic system has excitatory (+) and inhibitory (–) components; achromatic system is purely inhibitory (–). Responses of each system to short and long wavelength stimuli
are shown below. Simplified from Hamasaki (1970); Emily
E. Reid, delineator.

directly inhibit a green–red–absorbing cell through synapses between
the two photoreceptoral cells or indirectly through inhibitory nerve
cells (interneurons). To my knowledge, synapses between sensory
cells have not been demonstrated in any third eye, but the studies
conducted to date have not carefully analyzed the synaptic relation-

ships between cells and their fibers. Moreover, we need critical information on the presence (or absence) of interneurons. Lastly, mention should be made of the modifying effect of efferent (pinealopetal) impulses carried by nonmedullated (?) fibers in the frontal nerve (Morita, 1970).

The conclusions of Hamasaki (1970) are similar to those of the German school. Figure 73 is a simplification of his diagram of the conjectured relationships between photoreceptor and ganglion cells. The chromatic system is shown with its two components: a short wave-sensitive cell which exerts an inhibitory effect upon a ganglion cell, and a long wave-sensitive receptor which sends excitatory impulses to the same ganglion cell. The achromatic system is inhibitory at all wavelengths. Examples of responses of the two systems to stimulation with a short (342 nm) and a long (556 nm) wavelength are shown at the bottom.

For further aspects of the neurophysiology of the amphibian third eye, I refer the reader to the works cited and to Professor Dodt's forthcoming publication (Dodt, 1973). Moreover, I shall not discuss the electrical recordings from pineal and parietal vesicles of fishes (see Dodt, 1963; Morita, 1965, 1966a, 1970; Dodt, Ueck, and Oksche, 1971; Dodt, 1973). And, as stated earlier, I am placing the epiphysis beyond the scope of this essay.

I hope that I have now marshaled sufficient evidence to convince the reader of the photosensitivity of third eyes. Let us return to the consideration of their role in the lives of the animals which bear them. What use is made of their light-sensitivity?

Dosimeter of Solar Radiation.

The theory—call it Number 101—which Dr. Stebbins and I (1958) proposed for the role of the third eye in lizards is naturally our favorite. It was not completely original; one is always indebted to his predecessors for ideas and insights. We suggested that the reptilian parietal eye functions as a register of solar radiation. The designation *dosimeter* was first used by Robert Glaser (1958), one of Stebbins's doctoral students. It is a figure of speech. The eye does not count units of radiant energy (photons), but it responds to light with either "on" or "off" bursts of nervous impulses, as described. These neural messages pass to and through the epiphysis en route to neural centers, where we assume that they are integrated with impulses from other photoreceptors in the epiphysis and lateral eyes. Eventually, the endocrine system, especially the master gland of the body, the pituitary, is stimulated or inhibited. The flux and interplay of hormones which the endocrine glands produce modify in turn the behavior of the animal. The regulation of one important aspect of that behavior, to which we believe the parietal eye contributes, is the daily cycle of activity. This phenomenon is called the circadian rhythm, from the Latin *circum*, meaning 'around,' and *dies*, 'day' (Halberg 1959).

The circadian rhythm is an internal (endogenous) twenty-four-hour cycle with alternating phases of high and low physiological activity of an animal (or plant). Light is the principal external factor regulating the circadian rhythm. It has been called the *Zeitgeber*, meaning 'timer,' by Jürgen Aschoff (1954). A better designation offered by Professor Enright at La Jolla is *synchronizing agent*. The light cycle is a precise environmental clock by which we and other animals regulate the diurnal and nocturnal phases of our lives. By modifying the periods of light and dark, one can modify (entrain) the cycle of activity of an organism. The modification (entrainment) involves shift of the internal rhythm of physiological processes to correspond with the altered external cycle of light. Since this occurs in blinded animals–amphibians, for example (see Adler, 1970)—they must be obtaining cues from the *Zeitgeber* through other photoreceptors (extraoptic) such as those in third eyes. Not all amphibians have third eyes, of course, but they and other vertebrates have photoreceptors in the epiphysis and perhaps also in the brain (Dodt and Jacobson, 1963). Even though the extraoptic receptors do not give visual images as the lateral eyes do, they enable a blinded animal to detect light in the external environment and to determine the direction of its source. This information can be used in compass orientation (see Adler, 1970, for discussion). So far as orientation in relation to the sun is concerned, an animal probably relies on its lateral eyes, the dominant photoreceptors. And without them there would be only temporary value to sensing the presence and direction of light if, like my blinded Scelops, the animals could not see to capture food. On the other hand, whether the extraoptic receptors, in general, and third eyes, in particular, contribute significantly to the regulation of the circadian rhythm of an animal is an open question. We believe that in lizards, at least, they are important.

Parietalectomy.

The major defense of our theory rests on the effects of parietalectomy, the term adopted by Stebbins and me for the surgical procedure of removing a third eye of a lizard. To the word *parietal* we added a suffix from the Greek *ektome*, which means 'cutting out.' The ablation of the eye from a blue-bellied lizard is easily achieved by lifting the scale and skin above the eye, as described earlier, destroying the organ with a needle or tip of a knife, and replacing the skin and scale. The eye does not regenerate, and the parietal nerve degenerates. Parietalectomized animals (P) were compared with those (s) receiving a sham operation under both field and laboratory conditions (Stebbins and Eakin, 1958).

EFFECTS ON BEHAVIOR. Differences in behavior between P and s animals are subtle and demonstrable largely by statistical treatment of many observations. We found that P lizards in the field were exposed to sunlight for longer periods of time and at higher intensities of illumination than were s Scelops (Stebbins and Eakin, 1958). The former "arose" earlier in the morning and "retired" later in the afternoon, and they appeared to bask more than the latter. In an effort to quantify the differences between the two surgical types in the frequency of observing them, we recorded the number of P and s animals captured (or recognized by colored markers) on each visit to our study area in the Berkeley hills. In the total scores for the day each animal was counted only once, even though it may have been seen several times. This method was expected to give an indication of the relative numbers of the two groups exposed above ground. Our experimental population consisted of 373 lizards (272 immatures, 101 adults), half of them parietalectomized and the other half sham-operated. After surgery each animal had been returned to the precise place of its initial capture.

On 40 visits the score was in favor of the parietalectomized animals, on 15 in favor of the sham-operated ones, and on 8 the scores were equal. From October 23, 1955, to November 4, 1956, surgically treated lizards were seen or caught 703 times, the parietalectomized animals 409 times, the controls 294. The deviation from the expected 50/50 ratio is 4.34

times the standard error and is highly significant. The number of observations made on each surgical type has been calculated as a percentage of the total observations recorded on each visit to the study area (Stebbins and Eakin, 1958, p. 10).

Our graph of the results is republished here as Figure 74. Our conclusion that the parietalectomized lizards were "out from under cover" more than the sham-operated animals was supported by the study of Robert Glaser, who demonstrated (1958) a greater locomotor activity in Desert Night Lizards, *Xantusia vigilis* whose third eyes were covered with aluminum foil, than in unshielded animals.

Second, we reported a lesser "fright or escape reaction" in P *Sceloporus* than in s lizards. Stebbins and Cohen (1973) have just prepared a paper on a new field study of the effects of parietalectomy on *S. occidentalis* which confirms our observations. I am privileged to quote the following from their manuscript.

As noted in previous studies (Stebbins and Eakin, 1958) the field behavior of many (but not all) of the parietalectomized lizards was distinctive. They were reluctant to take cover and seemed strongly attracted to bright sunlight. Some individuals were pursued several minutes and, although wary of the noose, they tended to stay in the open and reemerged promptly from cover when frightened there. The senior author was able to predict a lizard's surgical type before capture with considerable accuracy. In a sample of 26 animals whose identity was unknown before capture, 21 were correctly recognized as to group. The probability of such a result occurring by chance is $P < 0.005$ (Chi-square test).

EFFECTS ON THYROID ACTIVITY. We found in our field study of P and s *S. occidentalis* and in laboratory experiments with the Desert Sand Lizard *Uma inornata* that there was a tendency for the thyroids of the experimentals to exhibit a thickening of the lining of the follicles (follicular epithelium) and a reduction in the amount of secreted material (colloid) in comparison with the glands of controls. The figures selected for publication (Stebbins and Eakin, 1958) were largely of *Uma*, who is not a member of my cast. So I recently unpacked the old slides which I had made of our field Scelops for some new micrographs (Figs. 75–78). I made the best match possible between two winter animals and two spring animals (parietalectomized with sham-operated). All were of the same sex

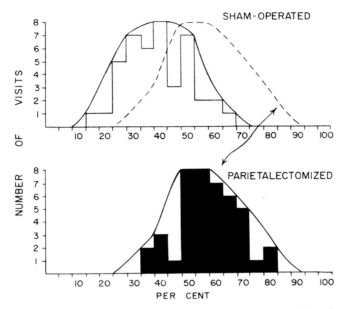

Fig. 74. Comparison of activity of sham-operated and parietalectomized *S. occidentalis* in field study. Number of observations made on each surgical type calculated as percentages of total observations made on each visit to study area. Percentage scores on horizontal axis; number of visits on vertical axis. From Stebbins and Eakin (1958).

and approximately the same size. The two winter specimens had been free-living in the study area in the Berkeley hills for a year or more following initial capture and surgery, and both were recaptured for histological examination on the same day in early November. Figure 75 shows a representative part of the thyroid gland of the control, Figure 76 a typical sector of the thyroid of the experimental. Both exhibit the inactive winter state of the gland which Malcolm Miller (1955) of our department of anatomy in San Francisco demonstrated for *Xantusia vigilis* and Daniel Wilhoft (1958), another student of Stebbins's, demonstrated for *S. occidentalis* (see Lynn, 1970, for other references). The diagnostic features are very low (squamous) follicular epithelium and uniformly dense colloid. The thyroid of the P animal, however, shows a slightly higher epithelium and a greater reabsorption of the secretion (more peripheral vacuoles) than that of the s lizard. Peripheral vacuoles give the margins of the colloid a bubbly appearance (note the upper follicles of Fig. 76).

The match of spring animals was almost as good as that of the winter pair. They were essentially alike as to sex, size, and length of postoperative time. The s animal was captured at the close of May, the P one at the end of the first week in June. Both exhibited the late spring, or breeding, condition of a Scelop's thyroid gland—very thick follicular epithelium and an abundance of peripheral vacuoles. In comparison with the control (Fig. 77), the experimental animal shows a discernible intensification of these features (Fig. 78). In some follicles of the parietalectomized specimen colloid is almost depleted; that is, it has been resorbed and utilized by the animal, and its epithelial cells are four or more times taller than the diameter of their nuclei, indicative of a highly active gland and suggestive of an elevated metabolism.

What is the evidence, the reader may ask, that the above anatomical features reliably signify the degree of thyroid activity? Most textbooks of endocrinology (for example, Turner and Bagnara, 1971) discuss the high correlation between the thickness of follicular epithelium and the appearance of colloid with the amount of circulating thyroid-stimulating hormone (TSH) from the pituitary gland. Thyroid disorders, responses to certain drugs (such as thiourea), and the like provide other forms of evidence. More modern studies involving use of electron microscopy, organ culture, and radioactive tracers give further documentation (see Feeney and Wissig, 1971, 1972). Stebbins (1973) has a brief paper in press showing that the highest uptake of radioactive iodine by *S. occidentalis* occurs in June, in correlation with the highest follicular epithelium and the greatest abundance of peripheral vacuoles. Iodine, as most readers probably know, is a strategic component of each molecule of thyroid hormone, and without iodine the gland cannot synthetize the hormone.

It was known from the study of Wilhoft (1958) that maintaining *S. occidentalis* at 35° C (the mean of the normal activity range) for several weeks leads to increased thyroid activity, and in a study I made (see Eakin, Stebbins, and Wilhoft, 1959) it was shown that this effect of temperature is mediated by the pituitary gland. These

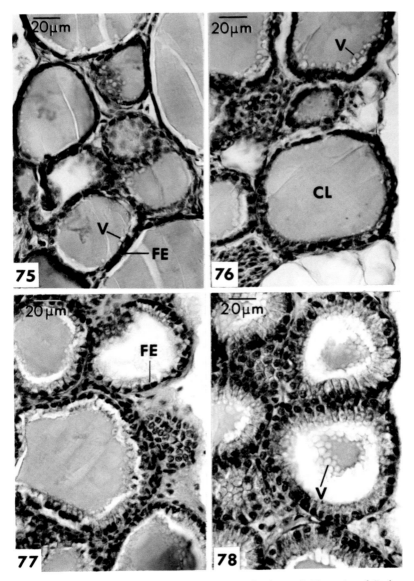

Figs. 75–78. LM of thyroids of *S. occidentalis* from field study of Stebbins and Eakin (1958). Figs. 75 and 76 show winter condition of, respectively, sham-operated and parietalectomized lizards; Figs. 77 and 78 show late spring condition of, respectively, sham-operated and parietalectomized animals. CL, colloid; FE, lining of follicle (follicular epithelium); V, vacuoles. × 360. Heretofore unpublished Eakin, Stebbins, and Tomlin.

observations led us to speculate that parietalectomized lizards, lacking their radiation dosimeter, spend more hours per day at their preferred temperature than normal lizards do. The stimulatory effect of increased radiation and the absence of impulses leading to inhibition release higher concentrations of thyroid-stimulating hormone from the pituitary. Greater thyroid activity (hypertrophy of the gland) results, and this in turn affects the behavior of the parietalectomized Scelop, as noted above. Parietal eye, epiphysis, neural centers (habenular ganglion and hypothalamus), pituitary gland, and thyroid gland are linked together, perhaps, in mediating the part the third eye plays in regulating the behavior of *S. occidentalis*.

EFFECTS ON GONADS. Near the beginning of this chapter I mentioned the study of Clausen and Poris (1937), who obtained evidence of heightened production of sperm (spermatogenesis) in the testes of *Anolis carolinensis* from which the third eye had been removed. The sex glands of these animals exhibited more sperm in the lumen of the canals (seminiferous tubules) and more cell divisions in the lining cells than those in normal lizards. These differences were exhibited by animals maintained under both normal and extended periods of illumination. The authors concluded that the third eye of a chameleon, responding to light, may inhibit sexual activity in some unknown way, directly or indirectly.

Paul Licht and Anita Pearson, who are near neighbors of mine in our Life Sciences Building, recently (1970) attempted to confirm the results of Clausen and Poris without success. They found no differences in histology or weight of testes between parietalectomized and control *A. carolinensis*, which had been critically selected so that the two groups were matched in size and which were maintained under carefully regulated temperature and photoperiodism (both long and short light days). They concluded: "the parietal eye does not affect testicular growth under short (non-stimulatory) or long (stimulatory) day lengths in the fall, nor does it appear to be involved in the testicular development that occurs independently of photoperiod at low temperatures." The differences in results obtained by the two sets of workers may be due to the fact, earlier pointed out by Fox and Dessauer (1958), that the controls used by Clausen and Poris were not of the same size as their experimental animals.

Stebbins (1970) studied the effects of parietalectomy on the re-productive tract of the Desert Night Lizard *Xantusia vigilis*. Animals from which the third eye was removed showed, in laboratory experiments, an acceleration in reproductive activity, in comparison with sham-operated lizards. Many experimental animals appeared to complete one reproductive cycle and to begin a second one by the end of the three-month experiment. It is noteworthy that P animals exposed themselves to light more frequently than did s lizards.

In a recent field study Stebbins and Cohen (1973) examined 82 P and 79 s Western Fence Lizards captured within one week near the close of April 1969. Surgery had been performed in the preceding fall and early winter. In the meantime the animals were free-living. The P females averaged heavier ovaries (by 40 percent) and higher ova counts (by 1.13 ova) than the controls. No differences were found in the reproductive activity of the males. The authors point out, however, that at the peak of the mating season it is difficult to detect differences in testicular histology and that there is great variation in the diameter of seminiferous tubules and in the height of the epithelial lining. They suggest that a future study should compare P and s males at some other season, such as "late June or early July after testicular regression was underway or in late fall or early winter during early stages of recrudescence" (onset of new activity).

EFFECTS ON BODILY TEMPERATURE. There was no significant difference in bodily temperature (more precisely, cloacal temperature) between parietalectomized and control lizards (Stebbins and Eakin, 1958). Our readings, however, gave only a picture of minute-by-minute thermal regulation. There are other aspects of this problem yet to be explored, such as total daily exposure to the optimal temperature, which are not reflected by our data. If we are correct in our observations that parietalectomized animals extend the length of time spent at thermal levels of "normal activity," the added period of elevated bodily temperature could have significant physiological effects.

MISCELLANEOUS PARAMETERS (FOR THE SAKE OF COMPLETENESS). On the basis of very limited study by Stebbins (in Stebbins and Eakin, 1958) life expectancy seemed to be affected by removal of the third eye. In one laboratory experiment he found that when food was reduced or eliminated P animals died before s lizards. Our field data and those of Stebbins and Cohen (1973), however, do not support the above conclusion, but in neither instance was the period of study sufficiently long for a satisfactory test of survival.

We observed no differences between P and s lizards in rate of growth, moulting, or pigmentation (Stebbins and Eakin, 1958). And no differentials in certain metabolic indicators (serotonin, monoamine oxidase, and acetylserotonin methyltransferase) were found between P and s Scelops by Quay, Stebbins, et al. (1970, 1971).

The Slow Worm Adds Testimony.

The European Slow Worm (also called the Blind Worm) *Anguis fragilis* is a limbless lizard whose tail is easily separated from his body at a breaking point. A doctoral candidate in Göttingen, Dieter Palenschat, compared the locomotor activity of normal and parietalectomized *A. fragilis* in relation to various parameters of illumination (intensity, wavelength, length of alternating periods of illumination and darkness, and such). I became aware of Palenschat's investigation through some remarks in the discussion section of Dodt and Scherer, 1968*a*. In correspondence with Professor Dodt I learned that Palenschat's thesis has not been published and that he is no longer active in this field, but Professor Dodt kindly sent me a copy of the summary of Palenschat's dissertation. The following findings of Palenschat, if confirmed, would support our theory.

1. Parietalectomized lizards lose synchronization with the *Zeitgeber* earlier than normal animals.

2. Parietalectomized Slow Worms exhibit considerably more activity than controls under illumination of a stated intensity.

3. Blinded animals (lateral eyes removed) with parietal eyes intact show "light-on" and "light-off" effects.

4. The activity of normal lizards is greater than that of parietalectomized ones in violet light, but in green light the reverse occurs (that is, controls are more active than experimentals).

5. The frequency of the activity cycles (circadian cycles?) is higher in parietalectomized animals than in normal ones.

The last words on the question of what value a parietal eye is to a lizard I give to my colleague Robert Stebbins, who was the initial

source of my interest in third eyes. He penned the following comment on my manuscript after a critical reading of it.

Parietalectomy leads to increased exposure to light and to the thermal
level of normal activity which, during the time of gonadal recrudescence,
can (may?) cause acceleration of the breeding cycle. I believe that the
"eye" of the intact animal prevents overacceleration during years when
there is an unusual amount of sunlight and warmth. It does so by inhibiting exposure during such warm, bright seasons.

And so the curtain falls on the last act of the play. But it rises again
for curtain call. The members of the cast are in a row across the stage.
Sceloporus does a few push-ups; *Hyla* inflates his vocal sac and makes
a series of croaks; *Entosphenus* wriggles joyously; the cilium waves
good-bye; and the author steps forward, makes a low bow revealing
the spot where he might have had a third eye (see Fig. 12), and says
to the reader:

THANK YOU.

Literature Cited

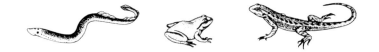

Adler, K.
  1970.   The role of extraoptic photoreceptors in amphibian rhythms and orientation: a review. J. Herpetol., 4:99–112.
Aschoff, J.
  1954.   Zeitgeber der tierischen Tagesperiodik. Naturwiss., 41:49–56.
Bagnara, J. T.
  1960.   Pineal regulation of the body lightening reaction in amphibian larvae. Science, 132:1481–1483.
  1963.   The pineal and the body lightening reaction of larval amphibians. Gen. Comp. Endocrinol., 3:86–100.
  1964.   Independent actions of pineal and hypophysis in the regulation of chromatophores of anuran larvae. Gen. Comp. Endocrinol., 4:299–303.
———— and M. E. Hadley
  1970.   Endocrinology of the amphibian pineal. Amer. Zool., 10:201–216.
Baker, P. C.
  1965.   Fine structure and morphogenic movements in the gastrula of the treefrog, *Hyla regilla*. J. Cell Biol., 24:95–116.
———— and T. E. Schroeder
  1967.   Cytoplasmic filaments and morphogenetic movement in the amphibian neural tube. Develop. Biol., 15:432–450.
Barnes, S. N.
  1971.   Fine structure of the photoreceptor and cerebral ganglion of the tadpole larva of *Amaroucium constellatum* (Verrill). (Subphylum: Urochordata; Class: Ascidiacea). Z. Zellforsch., 117:1–16.

Bleichmar, H., and E. De Robertis
  1962.   Submicroscopic morphology of the infrared receptor of pit vipers. Z. Zellforsch., 56:748–761.
Brink, A. S.
  1956.   Speculations on some advanced mammalian characteristics in the higher mammal-like reptiles. Palaeont. Africana, 4:77–96.
Brokaw, C. J.
  1972.   Flagellar movement: a sliding filament model. Science, 178:455–462.
Bunt, A. H., and D. E. Kelly
  1971.   Frog pineal photoreceptor renewal: preliminary observations. Anat. Rec., 171:99–116.
Burch, A. B.
  1942.   A microscalpel for use in experimental embryology. Science, 96:387–388.
Cameron, J.
  1903a. On the origin of the pineal body as an amesial structure, deduced from the study of its development in amphibia. Anat. Anz., 23:394–395.
  1903b. On the origin of the epiphysis cerebri as a bilateral structure in the chick. Proc. Roy. Soc. (Edinburgh), 25:160–167.
Clausen, H. J., and E. G. Poris
  1937.   The effect of light upon sexual activity in the lizard, *Anolis carolinensis*, with especial reference to the pineal body. Anat. Rec., 69:39–53.
Collin, J.-P.
  1969a. La cupule sensorielle de l'organe pinéal de la lamproie de planer. L'ultrastructure des cellules sensorielles et ses implications fonctionnelles. Arch. Anat. Micr. Morph. Exp., 58:145–182.
  1969b. Contribution a l'étude de l'organe pinéal. De l'épiphyse sensorielle a la glande pinéale: modalités de transformation et implications fonctionelles. Annales de la Station Biologique de Besse-en-Chandesse, Supp. 1:1–359.
Dalcq, A.
  1947.   Sur l'induction de l'épiphyse et sa signification pour la morphogénèse du cerveau antérieur. Arch. Port. Sci. Biol., 9:18–41.
de Graaf, H. W.
  1886.   Zur Anatomie und Entwicklung der Epiphyse bei Amphibien und Reptilien. Zool. Anz., 9:191–194.

Dendy, A.
 1899. On the development of the parietal eye and adjacent organs in Sphenodon (*Hatteria*). Quart. J. Micr. Sci., 42:111–153.

 1907. On the parietal sense-organs and associated structures in the New Zealand Lamprey (*Geotria australis*). Quart. J. Micr. Sci., 51:1–29.

 1911. On the structure, development and morphological interpretation of the pineal organs and adjacent parts of the brain in the tuatara (*Sphenodon punctatus*). Phil. Trans. Roy. Soc. Lond., 201:227–331.

Descartes, R.
 1662. De homine figuris et latinitate donatus a florentio schuyl. Leyden: Franciscim Moyardum et Petrum Leffen.

 1972. Treatise on Man. T. S. Hall, trans. Cambridge: Harvard Univ. Press.

Dilly, N.
 1961. Electron microscope observations of the receptors in the sensory vesicle of the ascidian tadpole. Nature (Lond.), 191:786–787.

 1964. Studies on the receptors in the cerebral vesicle of the ascidian tadpole. Pt. 2. The ocellus. Quart. J. Micr. Sci., 105:13–20.

Dodt, E.
 1963. Photosensitivity of the pineal organ in the teleost, *Salmo irideus* (Gibbons). Experientia, 19:642–643.

 1968. Das „dritte" Auge beim Grasfrosch. Umschau in Wiss. Technik., 2:54.

 1973. The parietal eye (pineal and parietal organs) of lower vertebrates. In *Handbook of Sensory Physiology*, Jung, R., ed., vol. 7, pt. 3. Berlin: Springer-Verlag.

———— and E. Heerd
 1962. Mode of action of pineal nerve fibers in frogs. J. Neurophysiol., 25:405–429.

———— and M. Jacobson
 1963. Photosensitivity of a localized region of the frog diencephalon. J. Neurophysiol., 26:752–758.

———— and E. Scherer
 1968a. Photic responses from the parietal eye of the lizard *Lacerta sicula campestris* (De Betta). Vision Res., 8:61–72.

 1968b. The electroretinogram of the third eye. Adv. Electrophysiol. Path. Visual System, 6:231–237.

————, M. Ueck, and A. Oksche

1971.   Relations of structure and function: the pineal organ of lower vertebrates. In *J. E. Purkyně Centenary Symposium* (Prague), Kruta, V., ed., pp. 253–278. Brno: Universita Jana Evangelisty Purkyně.

Dowling, J. E., and I. R. Gibbons

1961.   The effect of vitamin A deficiency on the fine structure of the retina. In *The Structure of the Eye*, Smelser, G. K., ed., pp. 85–99. New York: Academic Press.

———— and G. Wald

1958.   Vitamin A deficiency and night blindness. Proc. Nat. Acad. Sci. Wash., 44:648–661.

1960.   The biological function of vitamin A acid. Proc. Nat. Acad. Sci. Wash., 46:587–608.

Driscoll, W. T., and R. M. Eakin

1955.   The effects of sucrose on amphibian development with special reference to the pituitary body. J. Exp. Zool., 129:149–176.

Eakin, R. M.

1957.   Use of copper wire in noosing lizards. Copeia, 1957:148.

1960.   Number of photoreceptors and melanocytes in the third eye of the lizard, *Sceloporus occidentalis*. Anat. Rec., 138:345.

1961.   Photoreceptors in the amphibian frontal organ. Proc. Nat. Acad. Sci. Wash., 47:1084–1088.

1963.   Lines of evolution of photoreceptors. In *General Physiology of Cell Specialization*, Mazia, D., and Tyler, A., eds., pp. 393–425. New York: McGraw-Hill.

1964*a*. Development of the third eye in the lizard, *Sceloporus occidentalis*. Rev. Suisse Zool., 71:267–285.

1964*b*. The effect of vitamin A deficiency on photoreceptors in the lizard *Sceloporus occidentalis*. Vision Res., 4:17–22.

1965.   Differentiation of rods and cones in total darkness. J. Cell Biol., 25:162–165.

1968.   Evolution of photoreceptors. In *Evolutionary Biology*, Dobzhansky, T.; Hecht, M. K.; Steere, W. C., eds., 2:194–242. New York: Appleton-Century-Crofts.

1970.   A third eye. Amer. Sci., 58:73–79.

1972.   Structure of invertebrate photoreceptors. In *Handbook of Sensory Physiology,* Dartnall, H. J. A., ed., 7(1):625–684. Heidelberg, Springer-Verlag.

———— and J. L. Brandenburger

1970. Osmic staining of amphibian and gastropod photoreceptors. J. Ultra. Res., 30:619–641.

———— and F. E. Bush

1957. Development of the amphibian pituitary with special reference to the neural lobe. Anat. Rec., 129:279–296.

———— and A. Kuda

1971. Ultrastructure of sensory receptors in ascidian tadpoles. Z. Zellforsch., 112:287–312.

1972. Glycogen in lens of tunicate tadpole. (Chordata: Ascidiacea). J. Exp. Zool., 180:267–270.

————, W. B. Quay, and J. A. Westfall

1961. Cytochemical and cytological studies of the parietal eye of the lizard, *Sceloporus occidentalis*. Z. Zellforsch., 53:449–470.

1963. Cytological and cytochemical studies on the frontal and pineal organs of the treefrog, *Hyla regilla*. Z. Zellforsch., 59:663–683.

———— and R. C. Stebbins

1959. Parietal eye nerve in the fence lizard. Science, 130:1573–1574.

————, R. C. Stebbins, and D. C. Wilhoft

1959. Effects of parietalectomy and sustained temperature on thyroid of lizard, *Sceloporus occidentalis*. Proc. Soc. Exp. Biol. and Med., 101:162–164.

———— and J. A. Westfall

1959. Fine structure of the retina in the reptilian third eye. J. Biophys. Biochem. Cytol., 6:133–134.

1960. Further observations on the fine structure of the parietal eye of lizards. J. Biophys. Biochem. Cytol., 8:483–499.

1961. The development of photoreceptors in the stirnorgan of the treefrog, *Hyla regilla*. Embryologia, 6:84–98.

1962a. Fine structure of photoreceptors in amphioxus. J. Ultra. Res., 6:531–539.

1962b. Fine structure of photoreceptors in the hydromedusan, *Polyorchis penicillatus*. Proc. Nat. Acad. Sci. Wash., 48:826–833.

1965. Dissection and oriented embedding of small specimens for ultramicrotomy. Stain. Technol., 40:13–14.

Edinger, T.

1955. The size of parietal foramen and organ in reptiles. A rectification. Bull. Mus. Comp. Zool. Harvard Univ., 114:1–34.

1956. Paired pineal organs. Progr. Neurobiol., 121–129.

Feeney, L., and S. Wissig
    1971.   The morphologic and physiologic behaviour of thyroid lobes from newborn rats during short periods of incubation *in vitro*. Tissue and Cell, 3:9–34.
    1972.   A biochemical and radioautographic analysis of protein secretion by thyroid lobes incubated *in vitro*. J. Cell Biol., 53:510–522.

Fox, W., and H. C. Dessauer
    1958.   Response of the male reproductive system of lizards (*Anolis carolinensis*) to unnatural day-lengths in different seasons. Biol. Bull., 115:421–439.

Fristrom, D.
    1969.   Cellular degeneration in the production of some mutant phenotypes in *Drosophila melanogaster*. Molec. Gen. Genetics, 103:363–379.

Gibbons, I. R.
    1965.   Chemical dissection of cilia. Arch. Biol. (Liège), 76:317–352.

Gladstone, R. J., and C. P. G. Wakeley
    1940.   The Pineal Organ. Baltimore: Williams and Wilkins.

Glaser, R.
    1958.   Increase in locomotor activity following shielding of the parietal eye in night lizards. Science, 128:1577–1578.

Goette, A.
    1873.   Kurze Mittheilungen aus der Entwicklungsgeschichte der Unke. Arch. Mikrosk. Anat., 9:396–412.

Grell, K. G.
    1968.   Protozoologie. 2d ed. Berlin: Springer-Verlag.

Gundy, G. C.
    1972.   A comparative morphological study of the epiphyseal complex in skinks. Master's thesis, Department of Biology, University of Pittsburg.
    ——— and C. L. Ralph
    1971.   A histological study of the third eye and related structures in scincid lizards. Herpetol. Rev., 3:65.

Haffner, K. von
    1953.   Untersuchungen über die Entwicklung des Parietalorgans und des Parietalnerven von *Lacerta vivipara* und das Problem der Organe der Parietalregion. Z. Wiss. Zool., 157:1–34.

Halberg, F.
    1959.   Physiologic 24-hour periodicity; general and procedural con-

siderations with reference to the adrenal cycle. Z. Vitam.-Horm.-u Fermentforset., 10:225–296.

Hamasaki, D. I.
1968. Properties of the parietal eye of the green iguana. Vision Res., 8:591–599.

1969*a*. Spectral sensitivity of the parietal eye of the green iguana. Vision Res., 9:515–523.

1969*b*. Interaction of the slow responses of the parietal eye. Vision Res., 9:1453–1459.

1970. Interaction of excitation and inhibition in the stirnorgan of the frog. Vision Res., 10:307–316.

Harrison, R. G.
1907. Observations on the living developing nerve fiber. Anat. Rec., 1:116–118.

Heerd, E., and E. Dodt
1961. Wellenlängen-Diskriminatoren im Pinealorgan von *Rana temporaria*. Pflügers Arch. ges. Physiol., 274:33.

Hill, C.
1891. Development of the epiphysis in *Coregonus albus*. J. Morphol., 5:503–510.

1894. The epiphysis of teleosts and amia. J. Morphol., 9:237–268.

Holmgren, N.
1918. Zur Kenntnis der Parietalorgane von *Rana temporaria*. Ark. Zool., 11:1–13.

Jacobson, A. G.
1963. The determination and positioning of the nose, lens, and ear. J. Exp. Zool., 154:273–304.

Jarvik, E.
1967. The homologies of frontal and parietal bones in fishes and tetrapods. In *Problèmes Actuels de Paléontologie* (*Évolution des Vertébrés*), Lehman, J.-P., ed., pp. 181–211. Paris: Centre National de la Recherche Scientifique.

Kamer, J. C. van de
1949. Over de Ontwikkeling, de Determinatie en de Betekenis van de Epiphyse en de Paraphyse van de Amphibiën. Arnhem: G. W. van der Wiel.

Kappers, J. A.
1965. Survey of the innervation of the epiphysis cerebri and the accessory pineal organs of vertebrates. In *Structure and Function of the Epiphysis Cerebri*, Kappers, J. A., and Schadé,

J. P., eds. Progr. Brain Res., 10:87–153. Amsterdam: Elsevier.

1967.   The sensory innervation of the pineal organ in the lizard, *Lacerta viridis*, with remarks on its position in the trend of pineal phylogenetic structural and functional evolution. Z. Zellforsch., 81:581–618.

———— and J. P. Schadé, eds.

1965.   Structure and function of the epiphysis cerebri. Progr. Brain Res., vol. 10. Amsterdam: Elsevier.

Kelley, R. O.

1970.   An electron microscopic study of mesenchyme during development of interdigital spaces in man. Anat. Rec., 168:43–54.

Kelly, D. E.

1962.   Pineal organs: photoreception secretion, and development. Amer. Sci., 50:597–625.

1965.   Ultrastructure and development of amphibian pineal organs. In *Structure and Function of the Epiphysis Cerebri,* Kappers, J. A., and Schadé, J. P., eds. Progr. Brain Res., 10:270–287. Amsterdam: Elsevier.

1971.   Developmental aspects of amphibian pineal systems. In *The Pineal Gland,* Wolstenholme, G. E. W., and Knight, J., eds., pp. 53–77. London: J. & A. Churchill.

———— and S. W. Smith

1964.   Fine structure of the pineal organs of the adult frog, *Rana pipiens.* J. Cell Biol., 22:653–674.

Kitay, J. I., and M. D. Altschule

1954.   The Pineal Gland: A Review of the Physiologic Literature. Cambridge: Harvard University Press.

Kleine, A.

1929.   Über die Parietalorgane bei einheimischen und ausländischen Anuren. Jena Z. Med. Naturwiss., 64:339–376.

Kupffer, C. von

1894.   Die Entwicklung des Kopfes von *Ammocoetes planeri.* Studien zur vergleichenden Entwicklungsgeschichte des Kopfes der Kranioten, vol. 2. Munich: J. F. Lehmann.

Landis, B., and E. S. Tauber, eds.

1971.   In the Name of Life: Essays in Honor of Erich Fromm. New York: Holt, Rinehart and Winston.

Lerner, A. B.; J. D. Case; Y. Takahashi; T. H. Lee; and W. Mori
1958. Isolation of melatonin, the pineal gland factor that lightens melanocytes. J. Amer. Chem. Soc., 80:2587.
Leydig, F.
1872. Die in Deutschland lebenden Arten der Saurier. Tübingen: H. Laupp'schen Buchhandlung.
1890. Das Parietalorgan der Amphibien und Reptilien. Abhandl. Senckenb. Naturf. Ges., 16:441–550.
Licht, P., and A. K. Pearson
1970. Failure of parietalectomy to affect the testes in the lizard *Anolis carolinensis*. Copeia, 1970:172–173.
Linko, A.
1900. Über den Bau der Augen bei den Hydromedusen. Mem. Acad. Imp. Sci. (St. Petersburg), ser. 8, 10:1–23.
Little, E. V.
1914. The structure of the ocelli of *Polyorchis penicillata*. Univ. California Pub. Zool., 11:307–328.
Locy, W. A.
1894. The derivation of the pineal eye. Anat. Anz., 9:169–180.
Lynn, W. G.
1970. The thyroid. In *Biology of the Reptilia*, C. Gans., ed, 3:201–234. New York: Academic Press.
Mangold, O.
1931. Das Determinationsproblem. Das Wirbeltierauge in der Entwicklung und Regeneration. Ergeb. Biol., 7:193–403.
McDevitt, D. S.
1972. Presence of lateral eye lens crystallins in the median eye of the American Chameleon. Science, 175:763–764.
Meiniel, A.
1969. Etude préliminaire de l'organe parapinéal d'ammocete de *Lampetra planeri*. Arch. Anat. Micr. Morph. Exp., 58:219–237.
1971. Étude cytophysioloque de l'organe parapinéal de *Lampetra planeri*. J. Neuro-Visceral Rel., 32:157–199.
——— and J.-P. Collin
1971. Le complexe pinéal de l'ammocète (*Lampetra planeri*, Bl.). Z. Zellforsch., 117:354–380.
Miller, M. R.
1955. Cyclic changes in the thyroid and interrenal glands of the viviparous lizard, *Xantusia vigilis*. Anat. Rec., 123:19–32.

Miller, W. H., and M. L. Wolbarsht
  1962.   Neural activity in the parietal eye of a lizard. Science, 135:
         316–317.
Mizuno, T.
  1972.   Lens differentiation *in vitro* in the absence of optic vesicle in
         the epiblast of chick blastoderm under the influence of skin
         dermis. J. Embryol. Exp. Morph., 28:117–132.
Morita, Y.
  1965.   Erregung und Hemmung pinealer Neurone der Regenbogen-
         forelle (*Salmo irideus*) bei Belichtung des Zwischenhirns.
         Pflügers Arch. ges. Physiol., 283:R30.
  1966*a*. Entladungsmuster pinealer Neurone der Regenbogenforelle
         (*Salmo irideus*) bei Belichtung des Zwischenhirns. Pflügers
         Arch. ges. Physiol., 289:155–167.
  1966*b*. Absence of electrical activity of the pigeon's pineal organ in
         response to light. Experientia, 22:402.
  1970.   Wirkung repetitiver elektrischer Reizung des Pinealnerven auf
         die Antwort des Stirnorgans. Pflügers Arch. ges. Physiol.,
         319:R160–R161.
Nilsson, S. E. G.
  1965.   The ultrastructure of the receptor outer segments in the retina
         of the leopard frog (*Rana pipiens*). J. Ultra. Res., 12:207–
         231.
Nowikoff, M.
  1907.   Über das Parietalauge von *Lacerta agilis* und *Anguis fragilis*.
         Biolog. Centralbl., 27:364–370, 405–414.
  1910.   Untersuchungen über den Bau, die Entwicklung und die Bedeu-
         tung des Parietalauges von Sauriern. Z. Wiss. Zool., 96:118–
         207.
Oksche, A.
  1952.   Der Feinbau des Organon frontale bei *Rana temporaria* und
         seine funktionelle Bedeutung. Morph. Jahrb., 92:123–167.
  ———— and M. von Harnack
  1962.   Elektronenmikroskopische Untersuchungen am Stirnorgan
         (Frontalorgan, Epiphysenendblase) von *Rana temporaria* und
         Rana esculenta. Naturwiss., 49:429–430.
  1963.   Elektronenmikroskopische Untersuchungen am Stirnorgan
         von Anuren (zur Frage der Lichtrezeptoren). Z. Zellforsch.,
         59:239–288.
  1965.   Elektronenmikroskopische Untersuchungen an den Nerven-

bahnen des Pinealkomplexes von *Rana esculenta*. L. Z. Zell-forsch., 68:389–426.

———— and H. Kirschstein

1967. Die Ultrastruktur der Sinneszellen im Pinealorgan von *Phox-inus laevis*. L. Z. Zellforsch., 78:151–166.

1968. Unterschiedlicher elektronenmikroskopischer Feinbau der Sinneszellen im Parietalauge und im Pinealorgan (Epiphysis cerebri) von Lacertilia. (Ein Beitrag zum Epiphysenproblem.) Z. Zellforsch., 87:159–192.

Ortman, R.

1960. Parietal eye and nerve in *Anolis carolinensis*. Anat. Rec., 137: 386.

Owman, C., and C. Rüdeberg

1970. Light, fluorescence, and electron microscopic studies on the pineal organ of the pike, *Esox lucius* L., with special regard to 5-hydroxytryptamine. Z. Zellforsch., 107:522–550.

Palenschat, D.

1964. Beitrag zur lokomotorischen Aktivität der Blindschleiche (*Anguis fragilis* L.) unter besonderer Berücksichtigung des Parietalorgans. Dissertation zur Erlangung des Doktorgrades der Mathematisch-Naturwissenschaftlichen Fakultät der Georg-August-Universität zur Göttingen.

Petit, A.

1967. Nouvelles observations sur la morphogénèse et l'histogénèse du complexe épiphysaire des Lacertiliens. Arch. Anat., 50: 229–257.

1968. Ultrastructure de la rétine de l'oeil pariétal d'un Lacertilien, *Anguis fragilis*. Z. Zellforsch., 92:70–93.

Quay, W. B.

1972. Infrequency of pineal atrophy among birds and its relation to nocturnality. Condor, 74:33–45.

1973. Pineal Chemistry: In Cellular and Physiological Mechanisms. Springfield, Illinois: Charles C. Thomas. In press.

————; T. D. Kelley; R. C. Stebbins; and N. W. Cohen

1970. Experimental studies on brain 5-hydroxytryptamine and monoamine oxidase in a field population of the lizard *Scelopor-us occidentalis*. Physiol. Zoöl., 43:90–97.

———— and A. Renzoni

1967. The diencephalic relations and variably bipartite structure of the avian pineal complex. Riv. Biol., 60:9–75.

————; R. C. Stebbins; T. D. Kelley; and N. W. Cohen
1971. Effects of environmental and physiological factors on pineal acetylserotonin methyltransferase activity in the lizard *Sceloporus occidentalis*. Physiol. Zoöl., 44:241–248.

Rabl-Rückhard, V. H.
1886. Zur Deutung der Zirbeldrüse (Epiphysis). Zool. Anz., 9:405–407.

Ralph, C. L.
1970. Structure and alleged functions of avian pineals. Amer. Zool., 10:217–235.

———— and D. C. Dawson
1968. Failure of the pineal body of two species of birds (*Coturnix coturnix japonica* and *Passer domesticus*) to show electrical responses to illumination. Experientia, 24:147–148.

Reiter, R. J., ed.
1970. Comparative endocrinology of the pineal (a symposium). Amer. Zool., 10:187–267.

Riech, F.
1925. Epiphyse und Paraphyse im Lebenscyclus der Anuren. Z. Vergl. Physiol., 2:524–570.

Romer, A. S.
1945. Vertebrate Paleontology. Chicago: University of Chicago Press.

Roth, C., and R. Braun
1958. Zur Funktion des Parietalauges der Blindschleiche *Anguis fragilis* (Reptilia; Lacertilia, Anguidae). Naturwiss., 45:218–219.

Rüdeberg, C.
1969a. Structure of the parapineal organ of the adult rainbow trout, *Salmo gairdneri* Richardson. Z. Zellforsch., 93:282–304.

1969b. Light and electron microscopic studies on the pineal organ of the dogfish, *Scyliorhinus canicula* L. Z. Zellforsch., 96:548–581.

Salas, M., and S. Schapiro
1970. Effects of light upon pineal electrical rhythms. Fed. Proc., 29:325.

Satir, P.
1967. Morphological aspects of ciliary motility. J. Gen. Physiol., 50:241–258.

Schmidt, W. J.
  1909.   Beiträge zur Kenntnis der Parietalorgane der Saurier. Z. Wiss. Zool., 92:359–426.

Slifer, E. H.
  1953.   The pattern of specialized heat-sensitive areas on the surface of the body of Acrididae (Orthoptera). Pt. 2. The females. Trans. Amer. Ento. Soc., 79:69–98.

Spemann, H.
  1938.   Embryonic Development and Induction. New Haven: Yale University Press.

Spencer, W. B.
  1886*a*.   The parietal eye of *Hatteria*. Nature (Lond.), 34:33–35.
  1886*b*.   On the presence and structure of the pineal eye in Lacertilia. Quart. J. Micr. Sci., 27:165–238.

Stebbins, R. C.
  1954.   Amphibians and Reptiles of Western North America. New York: McGraw-Hill.
  1970.   The effect of parietalectomy on testicular activity and exposure to light in the Desert Night Lizard (*Xantusia vigilis*). Copeia, 1970:261–270.
  ———— and N. W. Cohen
  1973.   The effect of parietalectomy on the thyroid and gonads in free-living western fence lizards (*Sceloporus occidentalis*). In press.
  ———— and R. M. Eakin
  1958.   The role of the "third eye" in reptilian behavior. Amer. Mus. Nov., 1870:1–40.
  ————, W. Steyn, and C. Peers
  1960.   Results of stirnorganectomy in tadpoles of the african ranid frog, *Pyxicephalus delalandi*. Herpetologica, 16:261–275.
  ————, and W. Tong
  1973.   Epithelial height as a measure of thyroid activity in free-living western fence lizards (*Sceloporus occidentalis*). In press.

Stensiö, E. A.
  1963.   Anatomical studies on the arthrodiran head, pt. 1. Kungl. Sv. Vetensk. Handl., ser. 4, 9:1–419.

Steyn, W.
  1957.   The morphogenesis and some functional aspects of the epiphyseal complex in lizards. J. Comp. Neurol., 107:227–252.
  1958.   The pineal circulation in some lizards. S. Afr. J. Sci., 54:143–147.

1959*a*. Ultrastructure of pineal eye sensory cells. Nature (Lond.), 183:764–765.

1959*b*. Epithelial organization and histogenesis of the epiphysial complex in lizards. Acta. Anat., 37:310–335.

1960. Observations on the ultrastructure of the pineal eye. J. Roy. Micr. Soc., 79:47–58.

1961. Some epithalmic organs, the subcommissural organ, and their possible relation to vertebrate emergence on dry land. S. Afr. J. Sci., 57:283–287.

Stieda, L.
1865. Ueber den Bau der Haut des Frosches (*Rana temporaria* L.) Arch. Anat. Physiol., 1865:52–79.

Studnička, F. K.
1893. Sur les organes pariétaux de *Petromyzon planeri*. Sitzg. Kg. Ges. Wiss. (Prague), 1:1–50.

1905. Die Parietalorgane. In *Lehrbuch der vergleichenden mikroskopischen Anatomie der Wirbeltiere,* Oppel, A., ed., pt. 5. Jena: Gustav Fischer.

Taylor, A. N., and R. W. Wilson
1970. Electrophysiological evidence for the action of light on the pineal gland in the rat. Experientia 26:267–269.

Terashima, S.; R. C. Goris; and Y. Katsuki
1970. Structure of warm fiber terminals in the pit membrane of vipers. J. Ultra. Res., 31:494–506.

Thiéblot, L., and H. Le Bars
1955. La Glande Pineále ou Épiphyse. Paris: Libraire Maloine.

Tilney, F., and L. F. Warren
1919. The morphology and evolutional significance of the pineal body. Amer. Anat. Mem., 9:1–257.

Tretjakoff, D.
1915. Die Parietalorgane von *Petromyzon fluviatilis*. Z. Wiss. Zool., 113:1–112.

Turner, C. D., and J. T. Bagnara
1971. General Endocrinology. Philadelphia: W. B. Saunders.

Ueck, M.
1971. Strukturbesonderheiten der Anurenepiphyse nach prolongierter Osmierung und Anwendung der Actylcholinesterase-Reaktion. Z. Zellforsch., 112:526–541.

————, M. Vaupel-von Harnack, and Y. Morita
1971. Weitere experimentelle und neuroanatomische Untersuchun-

gen an den Nervenbahnen des Pinealkomplexes der Anuren. Z. Zellforsch., 116:250–274.

Wald, G.; P. K. Brown; and I. R. Gibbons
  1963.   The problem of visual excitation. J. Opt. Soc. Amer., 53:20–35.

Walls, G. L.
  1942.   The Vertebrate Eye and Its Adaptive Radiation. Bloomfield Hills, Michigan: Cranbrook Press.

Warner, F. D.
  1972.   Macromolecular organization of eukaryotic cilia and flagella. In *Advances in Cell and Molecular Biology*, DuPraw, E. J., ed., 2:193–235. New York: Academic Press.

Wilhoft, D. C.
  1958.   The effect of temperature on thyroid histology and survival in the lizard, *Sceloporus occidentalis*. Copeia, 1958:265–276.

Winston, R., and J. M. Enoch
  1971.   Retinal cone receptor as an ideal light collector. J. Opt. Soc. Amer., 61:1120–1121.

Winterhalter, W. P.
  1931.   Untersuchungen über das Stirnorgan der Anuren. Acta. Zool., 12:1–67.

Wolstenholme, G. E. W., and J. Knight, eds.
  1971.   The Pineal Gland. London: J. & A. Churchill.

Wurtman, R. J.; J. Axelrod; and D. E. Kelly
  1968.   The Pineal. New York: Academic Press.

Young, J. Z.
  1935.   The photoreceptors of lampreys. Pt. 2: The function of the pineal complex. J. Exp. Biol., 12:254–270.

Young, R. W.
  1970.   Visual cells. Sci. Amer., 223:80–91.
  1971a. An hypothesis to account for a basic distinction between rods and cones. Vision Res., 11:1–5.
  1971b. The renewal of rod and cone outer segments in the rhesus monkey. J. Cell Biol., 49:303–318.

Index